WORDS OF ENCOURAGEMENT FROM DR. ROBERT GILLER

I want you to try this diet. Even if you've never been able to stick to a diet before. Or even if you've never really reached your goal on another diet. Why? Because this diet is different. Here's how:

The Maximum Metabolism Diet:

- will speed your metabolism for *permanent* weight loss;

- will show you why eating too much fat, *even on a low-calorie diet,* can sabotage weight loss;

- will steer you away from the carbohydrates that are diet-busters and will direct you to *the correct carbohydrates,* the ones that help you burn fat and reduce hunger at the same time;

- will show you that *when* you eat is almost as important as *what* you eat in terms of controlling hunger, cravings and metabolism;

- will direct you to the *nutritional supplements* that will help your body reduce hunger and stick to the diet;

- will introduce you to the new psychological techniques that will help you approach dieting as a *positive* experience and that will help insure success;

- will show you how, by normalizing your metabolism, you not only lose weight and feel great, but also *live longer* by preventing the two most common causes of death — cancer and heart disease.

I think that the Maximum Metabolism Diet is the weight-reducing program you've been waiting for.

MAXIMUM METABOLISM

THE DIET BREAKTHROUGH FOR PERMANENT WEIGHT LOSS

BY
ROBERT M. GILLER, M.D.,
AND **KATHY MATTHEWS**

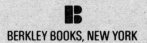

BERKLEY BOOKS, NEW YORK

This Berkley book contains the complete
text of the original hardcover edition.

MAXIMUM METABOLISM

A Berkley Book / published by arrangement with
Robert M. Giller, M.D., and Kathy Matthews

PRINTING HISTORY
G. P. Putnam's Sons edition published 1989
Published simultaneously in Canada
Berkley edition / April 1990

ISBN: 0-425-12180-1

A BERKLEY BOOK ® TM 757,375
Berkley Books are published by The Berkley Publishing Group,
200 Madison Avenue, New York, New York 10016.
The name "BERKLEY" and the "B" logo
are trademarks belonging to Berkley Publishing Corporation.

PRINTED IN THE UNITED STATES OF AMERICA

10 9 8 7 6 5 4 3 2 1

CONTENTS

CONTENTS

PREFACE

I want you to try this diet. Even if you've never been able to stick to a diet before. Or even if you've never really reached your goal on another diet. Why? Because this diet is different. Here's how:

The Maximum Metabolism Diet is dramatically effective. That's because it is based on the latest research in the field of weight control. The discovery that your metabolism can be responsible for weight gain and can be a major factor in encouraging weight loss was front-page news in the *New York Times* while I was writing this book. This information—on how you can alter your metabolic rate to achieve permanent weight loss—is the key to why this diet works. Once you read about the scientific background for the Maximum Metabolism Diet, you'll see how you can achieve your weight loss goals and you'll also probably see why you hadn't been able to in the past.

It wasn't developed in a laboratory. It grew out of my work with patients who wanted to lose weight. Many of these people had tried diets based on sound research principles but these diets, while they might have worked on mice or people in institutional settings, didn't work for them. After the success of my book *Medical Makeover,* many people came to me because they wanted to develop healthy habits that would prolong their lives and they wanted to eliminate minor symptoms—in short they wanted to feel great and live as long and as well as possible. But they also wanted to lose weight. *Maximum Metabolism* is the result of my work with these people. It really works on real people. My patients could fit it into their lives and so can you.

The Maximum Metabolism Diet is different from any other available diet because it does two things at once: It gives you a diet that works, and it tells you *how* to diet. Most diet books do only one or the other. They tell you what to eat *or* they talk about the psychology of weight control. In order to succeed you need both.

I know from my work with overweight patients that telling them exactly what to eat and when to eat it is only half the battle. You need to be able to deal with real-life dieting: restaurants, a spouse who's thin, a mother who pressures you to eat, job stress that won't quit and the habit of "fat thinking." You may be amazed to learn that what has been going on in your head could be partially responsible for your difficulty in losing weight. *Maximum Metabolism* will not only prime your body for weight loss, it will maximize your potential for success by helping you with the "inner game of dieting."

A final word: Prudence dictates that you consult with your doctor before undertaking this diet.

Part I

MAXIMUM METABOLISM: THE CONCEPT

Chapter 1

METABOLIC MISERY

Do you think that if only you could stick to a diet for a couple of weeks you could lose that weight? Do you think that if only you had more willpower you'd be thin, really thin, for the first time? Are you convinced that it's your own fault that you're overweight? Well, here are the facts culled from the very latest medical research:

Most overweight people:

- do not have to overeat to gain weight;

- can stick to the most demanding diet and not lose weight;

- can suffer very real and even overpowering physical cravings and crippling hunger on the wrong diet;

- can have lost weight successfully in the past only to find that the day comes when they can no longer lose weight on the diet that used to work for them;

- can sabotage the most effective diet by substituting the wrong foods—even though the substitutions may have fewer calories than the recommended foods.

If you're like most of my patients, you find these facts discouraging. They probably confirm what you already believe: that losing weight is difficult if not impossible.

Ten years ago most any failed dieter could have told you these facts were true but no one in medical science was listening. Today, however, the latest research has produced dramatic results for dieters and confirms what overweight people have been saying for years:

- "I can't lose weight no matter how strictly I diet."

- "I really don't overeat but my weight just creeps higher and higher."

- "I try to diet but I get so hungry that I just can't stand it."

- "I used to be able to lose weight but now nothing works."

If you recognize your own voice among these quotes, you should know that your problem is real and identifiable and we now know how to help you. We now know more about how your body works and how you can *make* it work to your advantage. These revelations are the best news dieters have had in years.

THE PROMISE OF THE MAXIMUM METABOLISM DIET

What if I were to tell you that losing weight isn't just a matter of willpower . . . isn't just a matter of eating a certain number of calories each day? Losing weight easily, quickly, safely and permanently is a matter of understanding that the problem is *not* just in your head; it's in your *body,* and your body can be changed. The way your body *works* can be changed so that you can lose weight, perhaps, like many of my patients, for the first time in your life.

If you have ever been on a diet and have failed either

because you haven't been able to stick to it due to overpowering cravings or because your weight loss was so slow or even nonexistent that you became discouraged and quit, then the Maximum Metabolism Diet could be the turning point in your diet history. It can help you lose twenty pounds in six weeks. Some people lose more quickly but you can depend on at least that weight loss. That might not sound like a dramatic weight loss but it is because it is really *possible*. What's more, the diet is not difficult and the improvement will be in overall health and energy levels as well as weight loss. Your weight loss will be *permanent* and any future weight loss will be even easier to achieve as your body reaches optimum metabolic balance.

The Maximum Metabolism Diet is the first weight-loss diet to recognize that each dieter has a unique biochemical makeup. To a large degree, what and when you eat determines how readily you'll lose weight. What and when you eat affects your metabolism—that most basic bodily mechanism that determines how fast and how well your body burns calories and produces energy. When you work *with* this knowledge, dieting is no longer a discouraging mystery.

Have you ever noticed that when thin people overeat nothing happens? That is, they don't gain weight. Maybe a pound or two but nothing to speak of. Almost every one of my patients has mentioned this with dismay. Well, the Maximum Metabolism Diet is the first diet that will make you more like a thin person. It does not rely on tricks to make you stick to a difficult diet; it relies instead on altering your body's very operating speed so that a sensible, delicious, highly nutritious, low-fat diet will allow you to shed pounds more rapidly than ever before.

I call my diet the Maximum Metabolism Diet because that's what it does. It changes the way your body works by accelerating your metabolism for quick weight loss, and it changes the way your body looks by helping you trim away stubborn fat that you may have given up on. It is a program geared to success: If you want to lose weight, only results count. In fact, it was this focus on results that inspired my diet in the first place. It began with the success of my first fitness and health program, Medical Makeover.

THE ORIGINS OF THE MAXIMUM METABOLISM DIET

Until the publication of *Medical Makeover,* my medical practice concentrated on nutrition and preventive medicine. I worked with people who suffered everything from elevated cholesterol to colitis to migraine headaches. *Medical Makeover* was inspired by the vast number of patients whose lives were impaired by fatigue, irritability, inability to concentrate and frequent headaches—ordinary complaints that many of us take for granted. These patients were usually under a great deal of stress and all of their complaints were exacerbated by that stress. I realized that their seemingly "minor" complaints were negatively affecting their lives today and were contributing to the development of serious disease in the future. *Medical Makeover* offered a program that helped my patients, and eventually countless readers, successfully cope with stress. It eliminated minor symptoms, restored vitality and good health and helped people improve their lives.

The great success of *Medical Makeover*—it was a national bestseller—brought me much professional satisfaction and, ironically, a frustrating problem. Many of the patients I had treated because they felt tired, run-down and overstressed also suffered from sweet cravings. Part of the Makeover program was geared to conquering sweet cravings and in fact I became well versed in the problems of sugarholics and chocoholics. I developed a very successful program to cope with these cravings. And because of my work with cravings, the nature of my practice began to change.

A new type of patient asked for help. These people exhibited the same symptoms as my former patients: They were tired, run-down, unable to concentrate and they suffered from headaches and irritability. But they were also overweight. So instead of treating a highly stressed run-down person I was now treating a highly stressed run-down person with a weight problem. I knew that I could help these people cope with their cravings but that was only half the battle: They wanted to lose weight. What made these patients more challenging was that they had invariably tried to lose weight in the past but had never really been successful.

I should confess right here that before I began to work with overweight people I harbored some serious misconceptions about weight loss. I thought that people who couldn't lose weight were emotionally weak, had no willpower and didn't exercise. I wasn't alone in this belief. A recent study has revealed that professionals, including doctors and even nutritionists, have surprisingly negative attitudes about overweight people. Over one-third thought that overweight people lacked willpower and 90 percent thought overweight people were self-indulgent. And these medical professionals are the very people who are supposed to be trying to help patients lose weight!

I am ashamed to say that I shared their attitudes. I thought there was no mystery to losing weight. I knew that there were low-calorie diets available and I thought all anyone had to do was to follow one until he or she reached the desired weight. How many times has your physician handed you a printed diet and told you to lose weight? This tactic has never been successful, though it is the approach most physicians take and I was among them.

What I've come to realize is that virtually every overweight person, whether ten pounds overweight or, like some of the patients I'm now seeing, one hundred or one hundred and fifty pounds overweight, has been on a multitude of diets. I should have realized that if those diets really worked, all these overweight people wouldn't be in my office desperately seeking yet another one! It took me a long time and work with many overweight patients to see that something else was going on.

Only after working with hundreds of overweight people did I realize that the stories they told me were *true:*

- Many of them did not overeat.

- Many of them did stick to diets without losing weight.

- Many of them had such powerful hunger and cravings that it was virtually impossible to stick to a diet.

- Many of them used to be thin and even though their food intake hasn't changed they've gained weight that they can't lose.

- Many of them gained weight after pregnancy or menopause, after crash dieting, taking diet pills or hormones, or stopping smoking, and then could not lose that weight.

- Many of them were as active or more active than any of my thin patients.

These people were telling the truth all along but their physicians just weren't listening—or worse, weren't believing them.

The stories of two overweight patients are typical:

Martina* had a diet history that featured all the most popular weight-loss programs. But the last time she was really thin—her ideal weight—was in grammar school. In

---

* In some instances identities have been altered to protect the privacy of my patients.

fact, Martina had a family history of overweight and through the years had become what she referred to as a "veteran of the diet wars."

Martina never had any problem starting a diet; she just couldn't stick to one. Her best intentions usually dissolved about the fifth or sixth day. By then, she'd usually lost a couple of pounds—enough weight to be encouraged that the diet was working. But also by then, she couldn't fight her sweet cravings any longer.

When Martina came to see me she was disgusted with herself and embarrassed. Embarrassed by her string of defeats, by the fact that she had never managed to lose weight. She is a successful sales rep in a busy sportswear company, a woman used to being in charge of her life and used to convincing others of her point of view. But why couldn't she convince herself that eating an ice cream bar was not in her best interests? She had decided that her problem must certainly be lack of willpower. She wasn't going to pass the buck and blame it on the diet. She'd tried a succession of diets and they had all worked—or at least would have worked if only she could have stuck with them.

Martina began the Medical Makeover program because she had heard it was a "no willpower" solution. When she completed it she felt better than she had in years. She was off sugar and sweets, off junk food, and she was drinking moderately. She had lost five pounds. She was feeling energetic and had even begun an exercise program. But she still had fifteen pounds to lose and wanted help. Every effort she'd made toward sticking to a low-calorie diet had failed when her overpowering cravings kicked in.

Julie's problem was different. Like Martina, she wanted to lose weight. But if embarrassment described Martina's feelings about her dieting, disappointment and confusion characterized Julie's. Julie had endless willpower. A lively divorced mother of two boys, she had managed to stick to the most demanding low-calorie diets imaginable while cooking nourishing meals for her children. When she came to see me she had just been on a modified liquid protein diet for a month. But she had lost only two pounds. By her calculations, that left twenty-two pounds to go and she would reach her goal in about a year. It was easy to see why she was discouraged.

Julie told me that no diet had ever worked for her. Moreover, whenever she dieted, she was hungry all the time. Even though she would stick to a diet that friends would find filling, she was constantly famished.

Why should it be so hard for her to lose weight? And why should it take so long? And why was it that diets that worked for others didn't work for her? She told me about the worst diet she'd ever been on. In fact, it was a popular, nutritionally sound program. Julie and a friend began the diet together. After two weeks, her friend had lost seven pounds and Julie had lost one, and that only by the third day.

Julie's diet history was different from Martina's. Her weight gain came later in life. After the birth of her first son, she never got back into her pre-pregnancy shape. She was always somewhere between eight and fifteen pounds overweight—not enough to be really troublesome as far as her health was concerned but enough to make her wardrobe obsolete and enough to depress her every time she went shopping for clothes, especially for a bathing suit. It was after the birth of her second son that Julie seemed to really settle into overweight. By the time she'd weaned him she had twenty-four pounds to lose and had given up even shopping for bathing suits. She had tried a number of diets over the past five years but nothing seemed to help.

When Julie came to see me she had almost given up on dieting. She was tired of hitting the "stuck needle," as she referred to her scale's reporting of her dieting plateaus. Julie had come to believe that something was wrong with her metabolism. She had had her thyroid checked and the results showed no abnormality. She wanted more testing done. There had to be something wrong. Most of all, Julie wanted me to know that when she went on past diets, she hadn't cheated.

What quickly became obvious to me was that there were a number of common denominators among people who were failed dieters. There was the problem of cravings. Some people craved sweets, others starches—but in either case these cravings were strong enough to sabotage the most determined dieter. Some patients noticed that stress of any kind made their cravings overpowering. Other patients told me that every time they went on a diet, they were hungry all the time. Still others claimed that they never felt full; they never knew when to stop eating. There was also the problem of plateaus. Some dieters would reach a frustrating plateau—they'd lose a few pounds but then their weight loss would stop.

The most troublesome aspect of all these problems is that every dieter I worked with believed that these were psychological problems. They were ashamed and confused because after failing at any number of diets they had developed a certain mind set: If only I had some willpower, some determination, I could stick to a diet and lose weight. Even people who had enormous willpower but who lost weight very slowly were convinced that it was somehow their fault.

I now know that there are biochemical problems and biochemical solutions for every failed dieter. Successful dieting isn't just a matter of willpower. The Maximum Metabolism Diet is the first diet to apply the latest medical research on weight loss to dieters like you. This is a "real-life" diet based on my success with thousands of patients. It's the first diet to solve your most troubling diet dilemmas in an effective, natural way by making your body work for you instead of against you.

Maximum Metabolism is a breakthrough in weight-loss programs because it is not a one-note theory: It doesn't depend on strange combinations of foods or severe caloric restriction or overdependence on a particular food group. Maximum Metabolism is a low-fat, calorie-reduced, totally balanced diet that works as a symphony. It recognizes that human appetite and cravings are regulated by a delicate biochemical balance between the part of the brain that stimulates the basic feeding mechanism and the various chemicals that affect it. Biochemical disturbances come from many sources—a lack of certain nutrients and overload of others, a diet high in sugar and caffeine, the presence of fat in the diet, etc. Maximum Metabolism is the first diet to recognize that foods are chemicals and that a delicate balance must be achieved to reduce hunger and speed weight loss.

The Maximum Metabolism Diet:

- will speed your metabolism for *permanent* weight loss;

- will show you why eating too much fat, *even on a low-calorie diet*, can sabotage weight loss;

- will steer you away from the carbohydrates that are diet-busters and will direct you to *the correct carbohydrates*, the ones that help you burn fat and reduce hunger at the same time;

- will show you that *when* you eat is almost as important as *what* you eat in terms of controlling hunger, cravings and metabolism;

- will direct you to the *nutritional supplements* that will help your body reduce hunger and stick to the diet;

- will introduce you to the new psychological techniques that will help you approach dieting as a *positive* experience and that will help insure success;

- will show you how, by normalizing your metabolism, you not only lose weight and feel great, but also *live longer* by preventing the two most common causes of death—cancer and heart disease.

I think that the Maximum Metabolism Diet is the weight-reducing program you've been waiting for.

Chapter 2

WHY CAN'T I LOSE WEIGHT?

B ARBARA AND PAM were college roommates. Each began
school at what she felt was an ideal weight. When they
graduated four years later, both were overweight: Pam by
twenty pounds and Barbara by sixteen pounds. Both began
working immediately after school and both dieted as well.
Within a year, both were back at their ideal weights. Ten
years later, Barbara has gained back those sixteen pounds
while Pam has remained slim. Barbara has dieted regularly
but after her initial success immediately after school, no diet
really worked for her. To the contrary, whenever Pam gained
a few pounds, she would diet it off within a couple of weeks.

Barbara is one of my patients. She told me about Pam
when she first came to see me. She confessed that she no
longer felt any eagerness to see Pam, who now lived in Los
Angeles. She couldn't help but feel that Pam saw her as less
than "successful" despite the fact that Barbara had a challenging job as project director at a major foundation. Barbara
was certain that her friend saw her as a "fat person" and

therefore "weak." Barbara's lament is among those that I hear almost daily:

- "Why is it that my friend can easily lose weight and I can't?"
- "Why is it that my spouse can eat twice what I eat and never gain?"
- "Why is it that even when I starve myself I don't lose weight?"
- "Why is it that as soon as I go on a diet, I'm totally starving?"

Ask most doctors or your slim friends and they'll be glad to tell you the two reasons you can't lose weight. As far as they're concerned, it couldn't be more obvious: You eat too much and you don't exercise enough. This brings us to two revolutionary findings that will change the way you think about dieting:

Overweight people do not necessarily overeat!

A recent article in a medical journal sums up the research: "Although it would seem that overeating is a necessary condition in weight gain, research has not been able to prove that, in general, obese people eat more than normal-weight people. Indeed, the evidence is impressive in its demonstration of the lack of clear overweight–normal weight differences in eating behavior."

Overweight people are not necessarily inactive!

At first I thought that if overweight people do not overeat, then perhaps their weight gain can simply be blamed on inactivity, though it was hard to see how that could tell the whole story. In fact, it's completely inaccurate. Research has shown that in general there is no difference in activity levels between overweight and normal-weight people!

How could this be true? It ran contrary to everything I had ever believed about overweight. And if it was true, then why *were* people overweight? Because if it wasn't just a matter of eating too much, or exercising too little, then I knew that there must be some other important factor in overweight, some factor that hadn't been accounted for in any diet I had ever seen.

METABOLISM: YOUR BODY'S MASTERMIND

My goal was to develop a diet that would work. Metabolism was the answer to my research and work with my patients. It was the factor that became a diet breakthrough. It was a simple answer with complex repercussions. Once I began to work with the latest research on metabolism—fine-tuning various foods and patterns of eating and supplements with my patients—I began to see astonishing results. People who had been stuck at twenty pounds overweight for fifteen years despite every effort finally lost that weight. People who had given up on dieting because of cravings and hunger at last stuck to a diet until they reached their desired weight.

Remember my patient Barbara? She was back at 123 pounds in eight weeks. She was thrilled to be headed for Los Angeles on a business trip. "I know this may sound petty, but one of my greatest pleasures will be to see the look of amazement on Pam's face when I visit her next month. I know she thought I'd never lose that weight."

What is metabolism and why does it matter in weight control? Metabolism is really the rate at which your body runs. It's easy to understand if you take a look at the concept of resting metabolic rate. The resting metabolic rate (or RMR) is the measure of how much energy, measured in calories, your body needs to do "nothing." Of course your body never does nothing; it's always circulating blood, breathing, digesting food, manufacturing chemicals at the cellular level and so on. Even when you're sleeping, your body is burning calories at your own individual resting metabolic rate.

Why does metabolism make such a difference to dieters? Because your metabolism regulates the rate at which you burn calories. If you have a fast metabolism, you use more calories to keep your body functioning. Therefore you can eat greater quantities of food without gaining weight. We've all been jealous of these people when we hear them boast that they can never keep any weight on: No matter what they eat they're thin. People with slow or sluggish metabolisms have the opposite problem: Their bodies have become terribly efficient, which is to say, it doesn't take many calories or much food for them to maintain their bodily functions. So despite rigorous dieting, it's almost as if their bodies are beating them at their own game: The less they eat, the less they lose. (And by the way, this isn't a matter of the "set-point" theory, which has been largely disproved.)

THE SEVEN ENEMIES OF MAXIMUM METABOLISM

Perhaps by now you've come to believe that your metabolism is to blame for your weight problem. And in the back of your mind you're thinking "Well, I'll try the diet, but if it's my metabolism there really isn't much I can do about it." Many of my patients have had this reaction when they first learn about the great range of metabolic rates. But the very point of my Maximum Metabolism weight-reduction program is that you *can* change your metabolism. But isn't metabolic rate inherited? Yes, it is. In fact, of the seven factors that influence metabolism, three are fixed—you can do nothing about them. They are:

- heredity (you inherit a metabolic rate just as you do hair and eye color);

- sex (the average RMR for women is between 5 and 10 percent lower than that of men—partly because women have a greater percentage of body fat than men);

- age (metabolism slows down with age)

The good news is that more than half of the seven factors that affect metabolism *can* be changed—to your advantage. I call these factors metabolic boosters. They are stimulating "brown fat" activity, taming the "hunger hormone," controlling stress and exercising.

Brown Fat Burners

One of the most important factors in the control of metabolism is something called "brown fat" and the latest discoveries about brown fat have created a real revolution in weight loss. Brown fat is a type of fat in the body, present in much smaller quantities than white or storage fat. Brown fat acts as a sort of "fat-burning factory," regulating the rate at which you gain or lose weight. Maximum Metabolism is the first diet that actually speeds up the fat-burning factory. It does this by accelerating the rate at which your body burns calories.

What do calories do? You probably know that they provide energy. In fact, at least 75 percent of the calories you eat go toward maintaining your resting metabolic rate, which we've already discussed. The other calories are expended in daily physical activity such as climbing a flight of stairs or walking. Of this last portion that goes to physical activity, an unknown but specific amount of calories go toward heat production or thermogenesis. This is where brown fat comes in. Brown adipose tissue, or brown fat, is the major regulator of thermogenesis. Brown fat is common to all mammals. It's located between the shoulder blades, the armpits, around the back of the neck and around the large blood

27

vessels in the chest and abdomen. Unlike white fat, brown fat contains a special protein that can convert caloric energy into pure heat.

What this means is that the more active brown fat a person has, the more heat he is able to generate and the easier it is for the body to lose weight.

Brown fat has been definitively linked to problems with weight loss. For example, one study found that overweight people tend to be less able to burn off excess calories. In this particular study, the metabolisms of lean people increased 19.6 to 25.3 percent one to two hours after eating, whereas the metabolisms of matched overweight people rose only 3 to 9 percent. To make matters worse, many scientists now believe that not only does defective brown fat burn calories less efficiently, it can also cause severe overeating.

It's this ability of brown fat that makes it the focus of the Maximum Metabolism program. Maximum Metabolism enables you to speed up your fat-burning ability to help you get rid of the white fat that we've all grown to hate.

How does Maximum Metabolism achieve this? Through regulation of the two factors that are known to slow brown fat activity: the fat content of the diet and the insulin levels of the diet. By the orchestration of these two factors we'll be able to maximize the activity of your brown fat and enable you to lose weight that you may never have been able to lose before.

Taming the "Hunger Hormone"

Recent research shows that a diet or an eating pattern that boosts the levels of the hunger hormone—insulin—in your blood can slow down your metabolism, can make you hungrier, can make it harder to lose weight and easier to gain weight.

Insulin is the hormone produced by the body that acts as a fuel regulator. It's responsible for getting sugar and fat out of the bloodstream and into the cells. Researchers have long been aware of that function of insulin. But there has been a very recent discovery concerning insulin that has had a dramatic impact on people who are struggling to control their weight. Insulin not only responds to what you've eaten; it also stimulates an appetite for more. That's why it's known as the hunger hormone. In an experiment conducted by Judith Rodin, pioneering researcher in the psychological and physiological factors in obesity, subjects whose insulin levels were stimulated by drinking sugar water outate the control group by over 500 calories when set loose at a buffet.

Insulin not only stimulates your appetite; increased levels of insulin can actually slow your metabolism and cause your body to store fat more easily. Therefore you will not only feel hungrier more often on an insulin-boosting diet, you'll also be more likely to gain weight. And if you're already overweight, you already have more insulin than you should in your bloodstream; the more overweight a person, the more insulin he has in his system.

The major insulin-boosters are sweets. The fact is that eating a candy bar can make you ravenous within a couple of hours. And, as most failed dieters know, sweet binges are self-perpetuating: A handful of cookies in the morning can spell disaster for the whole dieting day. But fats are implicated too: There's evidence that fatty foods can slow down glucose metabolism and create an abnormally high level of insulin in the body.

There's another aspect to how insulin works that once again proves that dieters' folk wisdom has more than a grain of truth to it. Many of my overweight patients have said ruefully, "I get fat just looking at food!" In fact it's now been proven that some people are what are called "hyperresponders." For these people, just the sight or even the thought of food can make their insulin levels surge, thus making them hungry. In an experiment reported in *American Health*, a group of people skipped breakfast and gathered at lunch to have blood samples drawn. Just before the samples were taken, an assistant brought a juicy, sizzling steak into the room. The hyperresponders showed a dramatic jump in insulin levels and therefore a dramatic jump in their level of hunger.

Maximum Metabolism is the first diet to regulate insulin levels by a careful pattern of meals and snacking. Fat consumption is as low as possible while still allowing for delicious meals. Sugar intake is minimal. Not only that, artificial sweeteners are banned. Most diets, by allowing artificial sweeteners, are planting the seeds of failure because such sweeteners may have the same effect on insulin levels as natural sugar. (This is another example of how focusing on calories alone is an outdated approach to dieting.)

Controlling Stress

Stress can also slow down your metabolism. It can make it more difficult for you to lose weight and more difficult for you to keep it off. Many of my patients have noted that they were doing well on a certain diet but that when a major stress entered their lives, they simply couldn't lose any more weight.

How can stress matter to weight loss? When the body is faced with stress of any kind—be it a traffic jam, an illness, an overwrought boss or even the stress of dieting itself—it prepares to respond with the fight-or-flight reaction. That is, the body releases antistress (adrenal) hormones, particularly norepinephrine. In a well-nourished, fit person, the body recovers quickly from the stress and goes on as before. The problem is that most dieters are neither well-nourished nor fit. Most dieters, indeed, most average Americans, are existing on what can be termed a "fast food" that depletes their reserves of micronutrients severely. Among these people—and certainly all my patients have been in this group—

the levels of norepinephrine have been severely depleted. When this happens, the body's fat-burning ability is impaired. They can no longer send the message via norepinephrine to the brown fat to function at maximum levels. At the same time, the lack of norepinephrine increases the insulin levels, which in turn increase hunger and fat-storing ability.

The Maximum Metabolism Diet is aimed at reducing the effect of stress on your body in two ways that will be described more thoroughly later in the book. The first is through an antistress formula of vitamins and minerals and the second is through exercise. Both these factors will help you fight stress and get your metabolism into high gear.

Exercise

There's no doubt about it: Exercise can be the most powerful factor in achieving Maximum Metabolism.

You probably already know about at least some of the benefits of exercise: It lowers blood pressure, it decreases the risk of heart disease, it decreases harmful cholesterols while increasing "good" cholesterols, it decreases the risk of osteoporosis, it raises energy levels and it's relaxing. In addition to these considerable health benefits, exercise is a major factor in weight loss.

We've talked about old-fashioned views of weight loss that strictly hold to the calories-consumed-equal-fat notions of weight gain. These theories maintain that a certain level of exercise would burn a certain number of calories. Thus you could burn off your chocolate bar with three-quarters of a mile of jogging. It turns out that this is an extremely limited understanding of the role of exercise.

We now know that aerobic exercise has a dramatic effect on your metabolic rate. In fact, exercise can help to encourage weight loss in three ways:

1. It increases your metabolic rate.
2. It increases and helps maintain lean body weight.
3. It causes enzymatic changes that facilitate fat metabolism.

While a crash diet can lower your metabolic rate, sometimes by as much as 20 percent, exercise increases your metabolic rate so that even if your diet remains the same, you will lose weight. Exercise also helps preserve lean body weight, which is a crucial element in effective weight loss. When you exercise you burn fat while you build or at least preserve muscle. An unbalanced, or crash, diet will force your body to lose a pound of muscle for every three pounds of fat lost. Finally, exercise stimulates your body to burn fat even after the exercise ceases. Your metabolic rate increases to the point that you continue to burn off calories at a high rate for up to two hours after an exercise session.

Exercise really is the linchpin of the Maximum Metabolism program. At the same time, I've learned that exercise can be a real challenge for some people. I've taken this into consideration in the Maximum Metabolism program. You will move into exercise gradually, as your body is ready for it. And you'll find that my supersimple exercise suggestions will make exercise easy to fit into your busy life.

WHY A SLOW METABOLISM IS NO LONGER HOPELESS

"So," you say, "it really *is* my metabolism. It's not my fault that I can't lose weight." In the past, people who were "diagnosed" (it was usually more a matter of guesswork than scientific analysis) as having a slow metabolism were, in effect, given a green light to obesity. It was believed that your metabolic rate was a simple matter of heredity. If you had a fast metabolism, you were thin and could eat with abandon; you were extremely lucky. If you had a slow metabolism, you were going to be fat no matter what you did so you might as well grin and bear it—and eat.

It is true that metabolic rates are closely linked with heredity, as well as with sex and age as we've just seen. But none of these fixed factors determine your metabolism exclusively. There are other factors that affect your metabolic rate and they are the basis for the Maximum Metabolism Diet. We're going to see how these factors become practical steps in your weight-loss program. They are:

- a balance of fat/carbohydrate/protein at each meal

- the number of meals eaten

- the timing of meals

- the use of vitamin and mineral supplements to control hunger and cravings and help you cope with stress

- the correct snacks eaten at the correct time

- an adequate number of calories each day (too few is as counterproductive as too many)

- an exercise program that is most conducive to boosting your metabolism and controlling stress

If you're like most of my patients, at this point you're asking, "But what about calories?" After all my work with overweight patients, my response has become: "It's not the number of calories but the type of calories that counts."

CALORIES ARE NOT MAGIC BULLETS

Most people fail at diets not because they overeat but because they do not have the average or ideal RMR. That is to say, most people are on a diet because they have a problem with metabolism in the first place. But the diet they are following is most likely based on the old-fashioned concept that fewer calories equal less body fat. But calories, though they've been given a starring role in almost every diet, are really best viewed as just members of the cast.

The Food and Nutrition Board tells us that the average American adult male of 154 pounds burns between 1,440 and 1,728 calories a day to sustain his RMR, and the average female of 128 pounds burns between 1,296 and 1,584 calories a day for the same purpose. So it follows that if you cut the calories needed to sustain your RMR, your body will be forced to find energy elsewhere—in stored fat—and you'll get slim. For some people this is the simple, correct solution. These are the people who have no trouble dieting. They go on a diet—cut down on caloric intake—and in a few weeks, they reach their goal.

But the simple, revolutionary basis of my Maximum Metabolism program is that metabolic rates are as different as fingerprints.

You know that hair and eye color differs dramatically among people, as does height and weight. But did you know that there's also enormous variation in metabolic rates?

For example, your metabolic rate could be 25 percent slower than that of your slim friend. So, though you both eat the same amount, you could weigh 25 percent more. Thus, if your normal weight is 130 and you have a slow metabolism, you could eat as much as your friend with a normal metabolism and wind up gaining forty pounds. The converse is also true: While your friend diets away an extra ten pounds effortlessly, you follow the same diet and lose nothing, or, as sometimes happens, you gain!

At first glance, this new information on metabolic rates is depressing. Indeed, it's a favorite excuse for people who have just given up on dieting: "I just have a slow metabolism so I guess I'll always be fat." If you rely on the old-fashioned concept of calories as magic bullets, you will be. But the Maximum Metabolism program will show you how to change the way your body works as you change your diet.

Chapter 3

MAXIMUM METABOLISM:
HOW TO ACHIEVE IT

"D R. GILLER, why is it that I'm eating the same number of calories I ate on my last diet but this time I'm losing weight?"

- "I never ate breakfast before but now that I'm eating Maximum Metabolism breakfasts I'm losing weight even though I'm eating almost the same amount of food that I used to eat every day."

- "It amazes me that cutting down on the fat in my diet has had such a dramatic effect on my weight loss—I'm three pounds from my goal. And I'm eating more than I used to eat."

- "I used to think that lots of pasta with red sauce would help me lose weight. But it never did work and I was always starving. Now I know why and I can hardly believe that I've lost twelve pounds so quickly."

If you used to believe that you were "stuck" with a slow metabolism that doomed you to overweight, these comments from four of my formerly overweight patients should encourage you. There *is* hope—no matter what the current rate of your metabolism!

Now you know what should be the most encouraging dieting fact you've ever heard: Though a slow or altered metabolism has been making it extremely hard for you to lose weight on conventional diets, we now know how to change all that. You may have been discouraged but the very fact that you're reading this book means that you have the one ingredient essential for success: willingness to try again. And this time will be different.

In this chapter you'll learn the principles of Maximum Metabolism. You'll also discover why so many diets may have failed for you in the past. And I promise you that, like most of my patients, you'll be relieved to find that the problem has not been you and your lack of willpower: It's been the wrong foods at the wrong times.

THE FIVE MAJOR METABOLIC BOOSTERS

Once you understand the factors that affect your own unique metabolism, you'll be able to work *with* your body to increase your metabolic rate and your weight loss. Here are the five major metabolic boosters that are at the core of the Maximum Metabolism Diet.

1. A low-fat diet.

You're probably well aware that a low-fat diet is an essential component of weight control. But if your understanding of the dangers of fat follows the old-fashioned concept of calories as magic bullets, then you could still find yourself cheating in a way that could sabotage your diet. Maximum Metabolism is the first diet to incorporate the latest research on the repercussions of fat in the diet and this information will change the way you approach dieting.

The time-honored belief that fat is "bad" for a diet is based on the caloric density of fats. That is to say, fats have far more calories per volume than protein or carbohydrates; an ounce of fat has more calories than an ounce of protein or carbohydrates. What this meant to many dieters in the past was that they played the game of calorie substitution and believed they could still lose weight: They would forgo the poached chicken breast at lunch and indulge in a small bowl of ice cream instead. If both foods had the same number of calories, they were doing fine. Or so they thought.

But we now know it's not just calories that count. There is increasing evidence that fats are uniquely fattening! It's as simple as that. Fat makes fat!

Fats are more readily stored as fat in your body, and they slow down your metabolism so you gain additional fat. It's a vicious circle. In fact, fat in your diet slows your brown fat activity and therefore your metabolism by as much as 25 percent! This is a huge slow-down in your fat-burning ability and you can see that, even if your caloric intake is low but your fat intake is high, you could be fighting a losing battle.

Not only does the fat in your diet slow your metabolism and make it more difficult for you to lose weight, it also makes it easier for you to gain! That's because the energy from fat is easily stored by your body as fat on your stomach, thighs, hips or wherever it is that your particular body tends to store fat. Carbohydrate energy, to the contrary, is stored in small amounts in the liver and in muscle tissue. It is rarely turned into body fat.

Not only does your body store fat as fat, it does it easily. It costs your body more calories to store carbohydrates: It has to make intermediate substances, a process that demands energy in the form of calories. One researcher has calculated that to turn 100 calories of carbohydrate into fat "costs" about 23 calories. To turn 100 calories of fat into body fat "costs" only 3 calories. In other words, fat can cause you to gain weight 20 percent faster!

One of the problems with fat reduction that dieters face is

that fats taste good. Nature intended it that way: If we're compelled to eat fats we'll be well prepared for starvation. The achievement of the Maximum Metabolism Diet has been to find the optimal balance between excess fat and good taste.

Barbara, a typical patient, said: "I used to think that a tiny piece of cheese was a good snack. I figured I needed the calcium even though the calories might be higher than I liked. I had no idea what that fat, added to the fat already in my diet, was doing to me. Not only couldn't I lose weight, I really felt sluggish. I'm amazed at how I can be satisfied on the Maximum Metabolism snacks of fruit and I've never felt so energetic. It's hard to believe I can eat this way and lose weight too!"

Many people are confused about the amount of fat in foods. How much fat does a steak really have? What about milk? Cottage cheese? How much can you eat? The Maximum Metabolism program has simplified the challenge of eating the right amount of fat to encourage maximum metabolism. First, following the menus in the back of this book will keep you on track. Second, when in doubt you can refer to the chart on fat content on pages 68–69. And finally, I offer a simple guideline: You can eat any foods that have a fat content of 25 percent or less. You can check food labels to discover fat content (see "Figuring the Fat" on page 70) and you can refer to the chart concerning fats in your foods. Remember that you must be scrupulous. Frozen dinners, for example, have 30 to 50 percent fat. And the difference between skim milk and 2 percent milk is huge: The former has 12 percent fat while the latter has 36 percent!

2. The right carbohydrates.

You know that complex carbohydrates are good for you. You know that they contain fiber, which aids in digestion and also helps prevent life-threatening diseases such as colon cancer. You also know now that carbohydrates "cost" your body more energy in the form of calories to digest than fats and are therefore a boon to dieters. Another bonus of carbohydrates is that they are high in bulk and therefore help to make you feel full. But there is one crucial thing you need to know about carbohydrates to make the Maximum Metabolism program work for you. All carbohydrates are not alike.

When the major food groups are discussed, they are divided into three groups: fats, protein and carbohydrates. Simple carbohydrates are the "diet destroyers": cakes, cookies, candy—foods that are comprised of lots of sugar and refined flour. Simple carbohydrates have no place in any diet, even one that isn't emphasizing weight control. You'll learn more about the dangers of simple carbohydrates in your first week on the Maximum Metabolism Diet. But for now, we need to make a further distinction among carbohydrates.

There are two types of complex carbohydrates: starchy complex carbohydrates such as grains, bread, potatoes, etc., and nonstarchy complex carbohydrates such as most fruits and vegetables. In the past, some diets emphasized the nearly complete elimination of starchy carbohydrates. This was when starches were viewed as "fattening." The pendulum has swung the other way today with many diets that propose carbohydrates as the perfect "diet food." The truth, as far as boosting your metabolism goes, lies somewhere in between. To achieve Maximum Metabolism, you need to cut down on the starchy complex carbohydrates and increase your intake of the nonstarchy complex carbohydrates.

I've had countless patients come to me with what I call the "pasta problem." They've followed the advice of recent diets and have cut down drastically on protein, particularly red meat. They have emphasized carbohydrates, especially bread, plain baked potatoes and pasta with tomato sauces. They should be losing weight but they're not. These are the people who gave me the mission to find the food combination that would allow them to have a diet breakthrough. It turned out that these people were partially right: They do need carbohydrates, but their emphasis was wrong. When they ate starchy carbohydrates—bread, potatoes, pasta, rice—they couldn't lose weight. When they switched to the right carbohydrates—nonstarchy fruits and vegetables— they began to lose dramatically.

This is one of the essential keys to the Maximum Metabolism Diet: Less starch equals faster weight loss.

There's another point to be made here: Carbohydrate cravers are really *starch* cravers. Starch is what slows down their diets. Broccoli is a high-carbohydrate food but have you ever heard of a carbohydrate-craver binging on broccoli? As Maryanne, a computer analyst, told me: "I was always able to lose a few pounds on a low-calorie diet. But I never seemed to get beyond a plateau weight that was about ten pounds over my goal—and I'd soon gain the lost weight right back. While dieting, I ate lots of pasta at night but never with cream sauces and my daily calorie count was very low. But to be honest, I always craved more carbohydrates: I was dying to have some bread with that pasta and sometimes I did.

"When I switched to the Maximum Metabolism Diet, I didn't even realize at first that the starches were so limited. But when I began to lose weight beyond my plateau weight, I knew something was different. I've now lost fifteen pounds and I know I'm going to reach my goal of twenty-five. And I've noticed that my cravings are completely gone."

The Maximum Metabolism Diet does not *eliminate* carbohydrates. It's a well-balanced diet that's easy to live with and you do need the vitamins, minerals and fiber of a richly varied diet. But I have changed the carbohydrate *emphasis:* lots of cellulose-rich carbohydrates and limited starch carbohydrates. In other words: Think fruits and vegetables.

An additional benefit of increased amounts of the right

carbohydrates is that you can eat more. For example, two cups of broccoli equals the calories and fiber of one slice of white bread. And there's far more bulk to the broccoli so you're going to feel full faster. You'll probably find, like all of my patients, that you've never felt so satisfied on a diet before.

The timing of your starch intake is also crucial. Breakfast is the *only* time that you're allowed starch on the Maximum Metabolism Diet. I've found that a morning starch boost helps to eliminate starch cravings throughout the day. Moreover it doesn't interfere with the accelerated metabolism that's our goal.

So two important keynotes of the Maximum Metabolism weight-reduction program are:

- *carbohydrates = fruits and vegetables*
- *starches only in the morning*

This approach has been the breakthrough that's allowed many of my patients to crash through their former plateau weights and reach their goals. The only starchy carbohydrates that are allowed on the diet are at breakfast. For the remainder of the day, you will have virtually unlimited cellulose-rich carbohydrates, including most fruits and vegetables. You'll find this combination of foods totally satisfying and your waistline will soon prove the effectiveness of a low-starch diet.

3. Timing and sequence of meals.

Have you ever dieted by skipping breakfast, having a light lunch (a container of yogurt perhaps) and then eating a late dinner that is probably larger than you'd planned because you're so famished? This is one of the most popular self-administered diets among my patients. They reason that because they're so busy during the day, they won't notice being hungry. They're correct about that aspect of their dinner-heavy diet. But it has two major flaws. First, it encourages a nighttime binge. Almost *all* of the patients who have tried this sort of diet confessed that on a few occasions they had lost all restraints by 10 P.M. They would gorge on cookies, pasta, ice cream, bread—virtually anything they could get their hands on. One woman told me that she ate a whole bag of frozen chocolate chip cookies she had put in the freezer to prevent her from snacking on them!

There's another major flaw to this kind of diet: It ignores the effect of meal timing and sequence on metabolism. In fact, researchers have demonstrated that eating fewer meals causes the body to become better at storing fat. Obviously, the body that is more efficient at storing fat is going to be a fatter body. Moreover, it will have more difficulty losing weight even when the meal pattern is changed.

The reason this happens is because irregular meals disrupt the ability of insulin, the "hunger hormone," to keep your metabolism running at peak efficiency. You'll have energy highs and lows, periods of extreme hunger and perhaps minor symptoms of headache and fatigue. And of course, worst of all for the dieter, you'll have trouble losing weight and find it much easier to gain.

Maximum Metabolism speeds weight loss with a sequence of well-planned, balanced meals that encourage an efficient metabolism. As Dora, a librarian, told me: "I find that I can eat *more* calories spread through the day than I did in the past and I lose *more* weight. When I had my major meal at 5 P.M., with virtually nothing before, I just couldn't lose. And needless to say, I was starving all the time! Now I'm losing steadily and I'm never tempted to snack at night."

Moreover, researchers have found that late meals contribute to weight gain. They can't explain why. They suspect it has something to do with the metabolic changes during sleep. They simply know that subjects who consume meals late in the day, especially after 9 P.M., will show a greater weight gain than subjects who eat earlier. This is regardless of number of calories consumed. This is why I recommend that on the Maximum Metabolism weight-reduction program, you never sit down to eat dinner later than 8 P.M. I've found that 7 P.M. is even more effective, though some patients simply can't eat that early. Whatever your schedule, make your dinner as early as is reasonable and be sure that your last meal of the day is not your largest.

4. Maximum nutrition.

I can't remind you too often that losing weight is not just a matter of *calories;* it's a question of increasing your metabolism so that *what* and *when* you eat is as important as *how much* you eat. Indeed, recent research has shown that a moderate calorie reduction is as effective and better tolerated for weight loss than extreme low-calorie diets.

For one thing, the weight lost at the beginning of such a low-calorie diet is not fat but water. It's quickly replaced and terribly discouraging for dieters, who are often prompted to stop dieting once the water-weight loss is accomplished and subsequent weight loss is negligible.

The other disadvantage of low-calorie diets is that if you consume fewer than 900 calories a day, you'll lose muscle tissue as well as fat. If you go lower than 900 calories, you'll lose even more muscle tissue as compared to fat. You'll lose weight, but it will be muscle and you'll actually be fatter than you were before the diet; the percentage of muscle will go down as the percentage of fat goes up.

The biggest problem with a severe low-calorie diet is that it can cause metabolism to slow down dramatically! In fact studies have demonstrated that a low-calorie diet can cause a 15 to 30 percent decrease in metabolic rates! The slowdown is even more marked in people who already have slow metabolisms—the overweight.

There's one additional drawback to diets that are severely

calorie-restricted: You simply can't count on adequate nutrition from a very limited food intake. Recent research done by Gallup has shown that the nutrition levels in the average American diet are, in most cases, deficient. For example, the typical woman averages only 61 percent of the RDA of vitamin B6, 61 percent of the RDA of iron and 78 percent of the calcium RDA. A severe caloric reduction can worsen these figures. And you'll recall how stress, including the stress of an inadequate nutrient level, can also slow down metabolism and sabotage a diet.

Obviously the challenge of a weight-reduction diet is to maintain optimal nutritional levels while promoting weight loss. Maximum Metabolism achieves this with carefully planned meals of adequate nutritional levels *and* a program of nutritional supplements. For example, because fat is such a problem, most cheese must be eliminated and therefore I believe calcium supplementation is essential. In the transition week of the Maximum Metabolism Diet you'll begin your program of supplements.

Finally, as you probably know already, severely restricted diets are severely unsatisfying. They're so unsatisfying that, while they might force laboratory rats to lose weight, they rarely work on people. As a University of Alabama study recently demonstrated, "Efforts to alter patterns of food *selection* may be more effective than attempts to modify eating behaviors." In other words, it's too hard to try to stop eating; so you might as well start eating the *right* foods instead. You'll feel satisfied and you *will* lose weight. And on the Maximum Metabolism Diet, you'll lose it even *faster* than you would on an extremely low-calorie diet.

5. *Regular exercise.*

Diet alone will help you lose weight. But if you exercise, your goal will be reached more easily and more quickly. If you exercise faithfully while following the principles of the Maximum Metabolism Diet, I promise you that you'll lose weight. It's that simple. Regular exercise is so important a metabolism-booster that you can lose weight almost twice as fast with its help.

A recent study of overweight women illustrates this point. This study made no effort to record what its participants ate; it didn't even put them on a diet. Nonetheless, women who began an exercise program lost weight even without dieting! The women who cycled lost 12 percent of their total body weight after six months; the women who walked lost 10 percent. That means that a woman who weighed 152 pounds and exercised an hour a day lost seventeen pounds. That's quite a demonstration of the metabolism-boosting effects of exercise!

Here are some of the ways that exercise helps you lose weight:

- Exercise burns calories.

- Exercise speeds up your metabolism for hours after you've finished exercising so that you continue to burn calories at a higher rate. If you exercise *before* you eat you'll increase your metabolism to an above-normal rate: you'll benefit not only from the calories burned during exercise but from additional calories burned after the meal.

- Exercise will depress your appetite by stabilizing insulin (your hunger hormone) and your blood sugar.

- Exercise makes you feel fuller when you eat by stimulating the production of hormones that raise the blood-fat level. These fatty acids circulating in your bloodstream make you feel full.

- Exercise will ultimately make it easier to maintain your reduced weight because it will increase your muscle mass. Because muscle is the major calorie-using tissue in the body (in opposition to fat, which simply *stores* calories), the more muscle you have the more food you can eat without adding body fat.

You probably know about the long-term benefits of regular exercise already. Perhaps the single most significant health benefit of exercise is that it strengthens your heart and reduces your risk of future heart disease. It lowers your blood pressure and decreases the levels of harmful blood fats such as triglycerides and other forms of cholesterol, while it increases the levels of the beneficial HDL cholesterols. In addition to these benefits, a recent study has shown that exercise can markedly reduce the risk of breast cancer and cancers of the reproductive system in women.

There's one final, and I think crucial, advantage to regular exercise: It makes you more energetic. Exercise brings more oxygen to the brain and makes you feel more alert throughout your day. I noticed this benefit of exercise myself when I first began to work out regularly. I found that I had more afternoon energy—when I had previously had a slump—and I was able to work in the evening if I wanted, something that had been out of the question before I began to exercise. Countless patients have commented on this benefit; some have even said that the increased energy and well-being they have achieved through regular exercise has been at least as valuable as their weight loss.

Despite all these proven benefits of exercise, I can't deny that many of my patients shudder when I first tell them they must exercise. As I'm devoted to exercise now and have seen the dramatic results of regular exercise in my own life, at first I really couldn't understand this reluctance. Until Barbara, a graphic artist who wanted to lose fifty pounds, told me: "You think exercise is just a matter of making up your mind to work out. It's like telling someone they have to diet and then they'll lose weight. It sounds so simple. But I'm fifty pounds overweight. Do you know how I look in a leotard? Do you think I would go to a gym, even if my schedule allowed? And I have three kids. I work freelance with no regular schedule. And I feel guilty enough about not being with my kids all the time: to take out time—which would have to come from my time with them—to exercise just isn't possible."

As I talked with other patients I began to understand that Barbara was not an exception. Exercise seemed just too complicated, too demanding, too "revealing."

But here's what Barbara told me the other day: "I never would have believed it. I'm just seven pounds short of my goal and I know that exercise made a difference. For the first week of the diet, I didn't move a muscle. I had had so many discouraging experiences in the past. But once I started to lose and to feel good, much to my surprise, I *felt* like exercising. And your suggestions about *how* to exercise made all the difference. I love the fact that I don't have to go to a gym and don't have to cut down on time with my kids. It's no longer a big deal to me. I don't think of it as an obligation. It's just part of my life."

When you read about the first week of the Maximum Metabolism Diet, you'll find greater detail on the three simple metabolism-boosting exercises I recommend and how to work them into your life. Once you've found the right exercise for you and your metabolism (swimming, for example, does not boost metabolism), I promise that you'll be a convert.

Chapter 4

Maximum Metabolism:

How to Stick with It

Jennifer, who works in computer graphics for a major television network, was late for her first appointment with me. "I could tell you it was the bus, Dr. Giller, but the truth is that I got cold feet and almost cancelled the appointment. You see, I know I need to diet. At 185 pounds that's pretty obvious. But I also know that I can't. I have no willpower. I can't stick to a diet no matter what it is. I'd really gotten to the point where I was convincing myself that 'fat is beautiful.' For some people that may be true but I used to be slim and it's hard for me to accept that I'll never be again. But I can't stand to fail again. I'm too embarrassed to even tell my friends that I'm on another diet. But Susan, another patient of yours, told me that I must come to see you before I gave up so here I am. I just want you to know that if this doesn't work it's not your fault."

Jennifer's story illustrates the second most common diet problem. The first, of course, is diets that don't work. The second is the inability to stick to a diet. In some ways it's worse than the first.

When a diet doesn't work, you pay for it physically. Not only don't you lose weight, but you also feel tired and irritable or headachy. You soon solve the problem by going off the diet.

When you can't stick to a diet, you suffer psychologically as well. You assume that something is wrong with you. Like Jennifer, you believe you have no willpower, no determination. And once you've failed, it's that much more difficult to try again. You're less likely to try another diet, more likely to see yourself as weak and liable to fail if you do diet again. It's a vicious circle.

I am here to tell you that there is a solution to your inability to stick to a diet. It's not all in your head, it's in your body. You don't fall off a diet because you're weak. You fall off a diet because it doesn't meet your body's biochemical needs. The Maximum Metabolism Diet will meet your body's needs; it will satisfy hunger and eliminate cravings. You'll succeed on this diet though you may never have succeeded on a diet before.

Listen to Jennifer today: "I know now that the biggest problem I had when I tried to lose weight was not me; it was the diets I was on. They just didn't work for me because I just couldn't stick to them. Now that I've lost twenty pounds I not only look like a new person, I think like one too. I know that dieting does not have to be torture. I know that I'm soon going to be slim again. I see people who haven't seen me in months and they don't recognize me. And even after they know who I am, they still don't recognize me! And that's because I'm more confident. That's what success does for you. I wish everyone who has ever failed at a diet, especially people like me who have failed at three or four or ten diets, would try your diet, Dr. Giller. It's not only for your body, it's for your mind."

I think I felt almost as much satisfaction with Jennifer's weight loss as she did. It demonstrated for me in the clearest possible way that my diet could work for everyone; that failed dieters are not weak people, they are simply on the wrong diet.

This chapter is going to tell you how Maximum Metabolism will be the one diet you will be able to stick to. It's all about what I call "diet insurance": a biochemical backup system that insures the effectiveness of your metabolic boosters. As your metabolism speeds up to help you lose weight, your "diet insurance" kicks in and eliminates the most common causes of diet failure: hunger and cravings.

If you are like most of my patients, you've come to think of the diet busters—hunger and cravings—as mysterious compulsions. You think you need to fight them with will-power. It probably never occurred to you that these impulses are indeed physical and can be controlled with very physical methods. This idea is at the heart of the Maximum Metabolism program: You *can* control your body. This book will teach you how.

HUNGER: THE #1 DIET BREAKER

- "I'm as ashamed of my appetite as I am of my fat. I could eat enough for an Olympic athlete at every meal and I'm always ready for a snack. Unfortunately I'm a typist and I guess that's why I'm twenty-five pounds overweight."

- "I'm only eight pounds overweight but I don't think I'll ever lose it. I'm always hungry. And when I'm dieting, I'm starving!"

- "My biggest problem with dieting has always been extreme hunger. I can usually stick to any diet until dinnertime. But when I get home I'm just so starving that I open the refrigerator and eat anything I can—cold spaghetti, slices of cheese, olives and mustard sandwich, whatever. I sometimes eat handfuls of cereal out of the box after dinner because I just don't feel full."

Do these stories sound familiar? Hunger is the most powerful of all diet deterrents. It's distracting. It weakens resolve. It wins the battle time and time again. The fact is, you can't diet successfully if you're hungry. The Maximum Metabolism Diet is geared to conquer hunger by tackling all the factors that contribute to this major diet downfall. Because it's too hard to fight hunger once it happens, the trick is to control it before it even begins.

Many factors affect hunger. Some of them have been recognized for a long time; others are recent revelations. The latest research demonstrates that the urge to eat and the sensation of fullness that tells us to stop eating depend on a complicated system of substances—some in the food we ingest and others produced by the body itself. As a recent *New York Times* article says: "The studies suggest that for people who are obese the exercise of willpower in weight control often means consciously opposing an inner chemical drive that says eat, eat or that fails to say stop eating." These inner chemical drives are the forces that we're controlling with "diet insurance." On the Maximum Metabolism program, we're going to employ the most effective methods of suppressing hunger and cravings so that you won't constantly be fighting your body in your efforts at weight loss.

How to Conquer the Hunger Hormone

As we've mentioned, insulin is also known as the "hunger hormone." It's the hormone that guides fats and sugars from the bloodstream into the body's cells. The surges of insulin working in the body after certain meals or snacks are recognized by the brain—the hunger center—and researchers have recently learned that increased levels of insulin make you increasingly hungry! This seemingly simple fact is the basis for one of the most effective aspects of the Maximum Metabolism Diet. It is the first weight-loss program that takes into account the role of insulin in the body. This single aspect of the diet could be the breakthrough that you need to lose weight, perhaps for the first time.

Have you ever noticed that you can be starving a few hours after a sugary snack? The popular misconception, at least among my patients, is that this signals a total breakdown of willpower: You give in to one sweet snack and you just can't stop. But this overpowering urge to continue eating sweets is a function of the insulin levels in your body. The increased levels of the hunger hormone after a snack tell your brain that you're even more hungry.

Does this make you a mere puppet at the mercy of insulin? Of course not: You simply need to learn to outwit your system. The exciting news is that if insulin increases your hunger, you can help to stabilize insulin levels, and therefore hunger, by eating the right things at the right times.

There's a bonus to this insulin-sensitive diet. It helps to free you from the vicious circle of overproduction of insulin. Once you're overweight, it's hard to lose weight because your body's cells become less sensitive to insulin levels. Therefore your body produces even more insulin in the losing fight to keep your blood sugar down. These increased amounts of the hunger hormone make you even more hungry and train the body to build yet more fat tissue. This is the phenomenon that results in adult-onset diabetes.

Maximum Metabolism is geared to avoid the factors that unduly increase your insulin levels. You'll fight insulin boosts, and therefore help conquer hunger, by following these five easy steps:

1. Reach for the "satisfaction supplement." That's the name one of my patients gave to guar gum. Guar gum is a natural fiber supplement that is readily available at your health food store. It has two beneficial effects in relation to hunger: It helps to regulate insulin levels and it helps to promote feelings of fullness. My patients have reported excellent results with guar fiber and I've made it an integral part of the Maximum Metabolism Diet.

   Guar gum is available in capsule form or as a powder. I

recommend you take two to four 500-milligram capsules three or four times a day. Most patients report the greatest effectiveness taking it just before meals. You can also take the powder by mixing about 1 teaspoon with a cup of warm or cold water (or juice) and drinking it. Guar gum usually facilitates bowel movements, though if you take too much you can become bloated and gassy.

2. Avoid sugar, the prime insulin booster. You'll work on this in the first week of Maximum Metabolism dieting and then throughout the diet with an eating program that provides flavorful fruit desserts and fruit snacks without resorting to the use of sugar or artificial sweeteners.

3. Eliminate caffeine, another major insulin booster. For those of you who think of yourselves as "caffeine addicts," you'll learn that you are indeed addicted and caffeine is doing more damage than you might have suspected to your entire physical well-being as well as your efforts at weight loss.

4. Eat balanced meals at regular times. Irregular meals— late meals, large meals—not only slow down your metabolism, they make you hungry by skewing your insulin levels.

5. Eat a high-fiber diet. The relatively high levels of fiber in the carbohydrates specified in the Maximum Metabolism Diet will satisfy your hunger both by helping to regulate the insulin in your blood and by adding enough bulk to your diet to make you feel full.

CRAVINGS: THOSE OVERPOWERING URGES

Hunger is that gnawing, empty feeling in the pit of your stomach. Cravings are those sudden obsessions with a particular food. As Barbara explains it: "I never had a real problem with hunger. And I always thought of hunger as a more 'honorable' problem for a dieter because I thought it wasn't your fault: you just weren't eating enough. But I really believed that cravings were failures of character. After all, what's my excuse for rushing out to the deli to buy some rum raisin ice cream at 10 in the morning? I never realized that there was a real physical reason for cravings. Now that I can control mine, I've lost eighteen pounds. And I don't feel like I'm always struggling to avoid even the thought of certain foods."

Cravings and hunger are really linked in many ways, but I've found that most of my patients experience them as two distinct feelings. Some cravers fit clearly into one of two groups: sweet cravers or carbohydrate cravers.

Recent studies have demonstrated that when and what you eat can have subtle and sometimes dramatic effects on your mood and behavior. Dr. Judith J. Wurtman is a cell biologist and nutritionist at M.I.T. and a pioneer in the area of cravings. Her studies have demonstrated that eating certain carbohydrates can raise the level of serotonin, a brain chemical associated with feeling relaxed, calm, sleepy, less depressed and less sensitive to pain. Dr. Wurtman has suggested that this explains why people binge on carbohydrates when they feel anxious or depressed. She continues: "It may also explain why high-protein, low-carbohydrate weight reduction diets usually fail. These diets induce a serotonin deficiency in the brain which in turn could trigger carbohydrate cravings to correct the imbalance."

The good news that we can glean from Dr. Wurtman and others working in the field of cravings is that these urges to eat certain kinds of foods are *biochemical* urges and not failures of character. Therefore our goal is to learn to fight cravings biochemically so we can stick to our diet and reach our goals. To do that you first need to determine the type of cravings you usually experience.

Are you a sweet or a carbohydrate craver? Some of my

patients ruefully admit to both. But many feel a distinct inclination to one or the other. There are some clues to identifying which "craver club" you might belong to. For example, women whose fat is mainly on the upper body—neck, shoulders and breasts—are more likely to have larger fat cells and higher insulin and glucose levels. This can lead to sweet cravings. On the other hand, women whose fat is mainly in the lower part of the body—abdomen, thighs and buttocks—are more likely to have smaller fat cells. They may be the carbohydrate cravers. And whether male or female, people who become tired, irritable and fatigued tend to be sweet cravers while those who become moody and depressed tend to be carbohydrate cravers.

Sweet Cravings

Many of my patients report that they feel sweet cravings as strongly as carbohydrate cravings. I think the big difference is that sweet cravers are truly addicts: sugar addicts. Their bodies have become addicted to the rush that sugar gives them and they may experience withdrawal when they can't have it. They have to be particularly careful to completely eliminate sugar from their diets to gain the most benefit from the Maximum Metabolism Diet.

Here are some of the "insurance tactics" I recommend particularly for sweet cravers:

• Take chromium supplements. Chromium is a natural mineral supplement that helps regulate sugar metabolism. Though the body needs only a small amount of chromium in the diet, it is difficult to absorb this amount from foods. Many studies have demonstrated that the average American is deficient in chromium. In fact, past dietary habits, particularly consumption of too much sugar, can create a chromium deficiency: The more sweets you eat the greater the possibility you have of a chromium deficiency.

I've found that chromium supplements can be enormously helpful to people who are prone to sweet cravings. I recommend that dieters take the trivalent form of chromium, in dosages of 100 micrograms, three times a day before meals. But it's important that you buy the right kind of chromium. I experimented with the various kinds when I created the Medical Makeover program and discovered that GTF chromium and chelated chromium will *not* be effective in controlling sweet cravings. Only trivalent chromium (usually available as a powder in a capsule) has been effective.

I think you'll find that not only does a chromium supplement help control your sweet cravings, it also helps you maintain stable energy levels throughout the day.

Susan, an exercise instructor, had always had a serious problem with sweet cravings: "I always thought of myself as someone with a sweet tooth. I simply couldn't resist sweets. I could control myself during the day, unless someone offered me a sweet snack. (I'm embarrassed to say that I was the kind of person who would sneak back to the receptionist's desk as often as possible if she had a box of chocolates.) But in the afternoon I told myself that I needed and deserved a sweet: it would give me a boost of much-needed energy for the afternoon. The fact that I was always dieting and that I could never, never lose that last ten pounds never stopped me. But I have to say that chromium made the difference for me. At first I thought it was psychological. But I went away for a weekend without my supplements and I really felt that old sweet urge again. This time I was able to resist it but I now see myself differently. After all, I finally have lost the ten pounds! But I can really see how your biochemistry can sabotage you and make you feel like you have no willpower. I think chromium has made all the difference in my dieting success."

• Reduce caffeine. Pat, a commodities trader, told me that she thought she'd never be able to live without coffee. But, as she was desperate to lose weight and had been unsuccessful at every diet she'd ever tried, she was willing to try to kick her six-cup-a-day habit. She was amazed that not only did she "stay awake all day," she felt more energetic than ever and "I finally lost ten pounds and I really think that being caffeine-free made a difference. I always felt like I was having peaks and valleys before. Now I'm on an even keel and that feeling of control has made it much easier to diet."

Remember when we saw the havoc that overproduction of insulin can cause? It makes you increasingly hungry and therefore harder to resist cravings of any kind. Caffeine stimulates the body to release insulin. The first reaction your body experiences is a boost of energy, but this is quickly followed by a slump that can leave you not only tired and irritable but also famished. It can be very hard to resist the temptation of a sweet snack in this condition. I'll tell you more about the dangers of caffeine when we discuss the first week of your Maximum Metabolism program, but for now it's enough to know that reducing the caffeine in your diet is going to help eliminate your sweet cravings once and for all.

• Eat regular meals at regular times. Once again, we're pointing the finger at insulin as a prime diet breaker. I've found that many of my patients who have failed at dieting in the past are people who have highly irregular eating patterns: usually no breakfast, a light lunch such as a container of yogurt, then more and more snacks and fatty foods as the day wears on and their hunger increases. Sometimes they make it to a light dinner—only to indulge in a carton of ice cream for dessert.

There are two problems with this erratic meal pattern. First, if you eat this way you tend to become dependent on quick fixes throughout the day in a desperate effort to boost your blood sugar. Your quick fix might be a cup of coffee, or three or four, or a candy bar or cookie. Whatever it is, you can be sure it's not going to help you lose weight. In addition, while the quick fix will temporarily boost your blood sugar and give you a rush of energy, it will then make you pay for that surge of energy with a slump that will make you feel tired and irritable later on. Worst of all from the dieting point of view, the quick fix will boost your insulin levels. And you now know what that means: hunger!

The second problem with erratic eating is that people seem to gain more weight on fewer calories. How could this be? Well, it seems that long periods between adequate meals instructs the metabolism to gear up for starvation: When the meal finally arrives, its calories are stored more quickly and permanently than the same calories consumed over a longer period of time. Gordon Ball, a behavioral therapist, found that the amount eaten at a meal is related not to the size of the previous meal, but to the interval between meals. A long interval means bigger amounts. If a rat eats his whole day's ration at once, his stomach and intestines expand, he absorbs his food 40 percent faster, and he becomes fatter, calorie for calorie, than a rat eating regular meals of regular size. It seems that this pattern also holds true for people. Moreover, people who consume most of their calories at one meal usually do so at night. For reasons that researchers have yet to discover, late meals are stored more readily as fat than early meals. A fascinating experiment demonstrated that if you eat all your daily calories at one sitting, a morning meal will result in weight loss; a midday meal will cause your weight to remain stable; and a late-night meal will cause you to gain weight.

- Snack on fruits. As you're well aware by now, the fluctuation of sugar in the blood and the surges in your levels of insulin cause hunger. To help eliminate these surges, I suggest that you have two fruit snacks a day. Fructose, the natural sugar in fruit, is metabolized more slowly than refined sugar and so will help to stabilize your blood sugar. You can have any fruit on the list of acceptable fruits (p. 105) twice a day. Most of my patients have a fruit snack mid-morning and mid-afternoon.

Carbohydrate Cravings

Most of today's diet research has focused on carbohydrate cravers. We now know that there is a hormone, serotonin, that is produced as a direct result of carbohydrate ingestion. Serotonin has a calming effect on the body. The lack of serotonin causes agitation. It is believed that some people have a naturally low level of serotonin and, in an effort to compensate for that deficiency, they crave carbohydrates. As I mentioned earlier, Dr. Judith Wurtman has demonstrated how the calming effect of serotonin can explain why people binge on carbohydrates when they feel anxious or depressed.

It's this craving for carbohydrates that probably spelled failure for so many people who followed the high-protein low-carbohydrate diets of the past. Dieters would feel such a powerful physiological urge for carbohydrates that they simply couldn't stick to the diet. Or they would binge on high-protein foods such as cottage cheese or meat, which contained so much fat and calories that it would slow down their metabolism to the point where no matter how few calories they consumed, they couldn't lose weight. Many of my patients have had dismal experiences with such high-protein diets in the past.

The Maximum Metabolism Diet is geared to fight carbohydrate cravings, while still promoting the accelerated metabolic rate that will insure weight loss. It does this in two ways:

• Tryptophan. Tryptophan is a natural supplement—an amino acid—that can effectively satisfy the body's cravings for carbohydrates. Tryptophan is converted to serotonin in the brain and so "tricks" the body into thinking it has ingested a carbohydrate. One study at the University of Lausanne in Switzerland found that patients who took tryptophan supplements while on a reducing diet lost more weight than patients taking a placebo on the same diet. The tryptophan reduced appetite and hence food intake. My patients have reported great success with tryptophan. One man told me that the only thing that stands between him and a cheese coffee cake at 10 in the morning is his supply of L-tryptophan.

I recommend taking L-tryptophan in doses of 125 milligrams between meals. My patients have the best success taking it between meals with their fruit snack.

• The Maximum Metabolism breakfast. As I've said before, one of the keys to the success of Maximum Metabolism is its emphasis on the right carbohydrates. We now know that certain starches can have a tendency to slow down metabolism, making it more difficult for you to lose weight. But it's also true that certain starches can satisfy the body's craving for carbohydrates. The Maximum Metabolism solution is a breakfast that allows certain starches—low in fat and in limited amounts—first thing in the morning. This amount of starch in the morning stimulates just the right amount of tryptophan to satisfy cravings but not enough to interfere with the increased metabolism that spurs weight loss. I recommend that all dieters, whether or not they think of themselves as carbohydrate-cravers, have this breakfast.

Part II

MAXIMUM METABOLISM: THE DIET

Chapter 5

Getting Started: the maximum metabolism basics

Tᴴɪꜱ ᴡᴇᴇᴋ ᴡɪʟʟ signal the beginning of a new way of life for you.

Your first goal is to prime your body for maximum weight loss in the weeks to come. You *are* going to get your body into the best possible shape to succeed with your Maximum Metabolism Diet. You *are* going to eliminate those factors in your life and your diet that are slowing your metabolism and preventing you from losing weight. You *are* going to incorporate some new habits into your life. These new habits will involve some simple changes in your day-to-day routine. By making these changes, you'll improve your overall health, energy level and psychological commitment to the diet.

What follows are the basic principles of the Maximum Metabolism Diet and how you're going to apply them. The actual diet and menus will follow at the end of the book.

THE SEVEN BASIC GOALS OF THE MAXIMUM METABOLISM DIET

In my years of working with overweight patients I've learned a great deal about what doesn't work as far as diets are concerned. My patients have told me time and time again that they are discouraged by complicated diets. They don't want to have to weigh food. They don't want to have to look up calories. They don't want to have to master a detailed system of "food exchanges." They just want to lose weight.

With that in mind I've tried to make the Maximum Metabolism Diet as simple as possible. If you follow the basic principles presented in this chapter, you will succeed on the diet. Some people need and want more detailed menu and recipe suggestions, so I've included them too. But the core of the diet is the principles that follow.

I suggest that you begin the diet on a weekend when you'll have time to adjust to your new patterns of eating, thinking and planning. It's best to choose a weekend that isn't busy; one that doesn't include any entertaining or visiting. That way, you'll be able to focus on adopting your new habits without the pressures and distractions of dealing with other people.

GOAL 1: Reduce the Fat in Your Diet

You already know that fat slows down your metabolism. Remember that one of the basic principles of the Maximum Metabolism Diet is "fat makes fat." So your first goal on the diet is to reduce the amount of fat in your diet by as much as possible. Don't worry about not getting enough fat; there's enough natural fat in chicken and even fish to fulfill your nutritional needs.

Here are the items you must eliminate from your diet:

avocado	luncheon meats
butter	margarine
cheese[1]	mayonnaise
chocolate	nuts[3]
coconut	oils[4]
cream sauces	peanut butter
eggs	red meat
fried foods	seeds
ice cream	shortenings
junk foods[2]	whole milk

[1] With one or two exceptions, noted in the recipes.
[2] Including all prepared baked goods, potato chips, etc.
[3] All types, including dry-roasted.
[4] Except olive oil.

Of course there might be a time or two, after you've achieved your target weight, when you'll have a steak or a hamburger. But, if you're like most of my patients, you'll probably find that by the time you do have it, it will have lost its allure. The same with fried foods and cream sauces and junk foods. You'll be amazed at how terrible these things will taste if you try them a few months from now. To be honest, I can't promise you that you'll totally lose your taste for ice cream, but the good news is that the time will come when you'll be able to have some ice cream, enjoy it and that will be the end of it. You'll be eating like a thin person.

Here is a chart that you'll find useful in assessing the fat content of various foods. On the Maximum Metabolism Diet you should choose foods with less than 25 percent fat content.

Where Your Fat Comes From

Food	Serving Size	Grams of Fat (and Types)*	Percentage of Calories from Fats
DAIRY & EGGS			
Swiss or Cheddar cheese	1 oz.	9	69%
Cottage cheese	1 cup	10	39%
Cottage cheese, lowfat	1 cup	2	12%
Whole milk	1 cup	8	48%
Lowfat milk (2%)	1 cup	5	37%
Skim milk	1 cup	.4	5%
Half-and-half	1 cup	28	80%
Yogurt, lowfat	8 oz.	2–4	10–25%
Ice cream	4 oz.	10–20	50–65%
Butter	1 Tbsp.	11.5	100%
Egg	1	6	75%
MEAT & FISH			
Beef, pork, or lamb, cooked,			
with visible fat	3 oz.	12–25	50–70%
all visible fat trimmed	3 oz.	5–12	30–50%
Sausage, pork, cooked	3 oz.	36	85%
Frankfurter, beef	1	15	79%
Chicken, roasted			
dark meat, with skin	3 oz.	13	55%
light meat, no skin	3 oz.	4	23%
Fish, fresh, broiled*	3 oz.	4–8	20–35%
FRUIT & VEGETABLES			
Avocado	1	37	90%
Others	1	0–1	0–8%
NUTS			
Peanuts	1/2 cup	36	75%
Pecans	1/2 cup	42	90%

Food	Serving Size	Grams of Fat (and Types)*	Percentage of Calories from Fats
GRAINS			
Bread	1 slice	1	13%
Spaghetti, cooked	1 cup	1	5%
Rice, cooked	1 cup	—	—
MISCELLANEOUS			
Coconut or palm oil	1 Tbsp.	14	100%
Other vegetable oils	1 Tbsp.	14	100%
Margarine	1 Tbsp.	11.5	100%
Potato chips	10	8	62%
Doughnut	1	6	54%
Chocolate bar, milk	1 oz.	9	56%
Mayonnaise	1 Tbsp.	11	99%

* Except the following high-fat fishes: anchovy, bonito, crab cakes, mackerel, pompano, sardines, tuna in oil, yellowtail.

* "Fat in Your Diet." Reprinted by permission of: *University of California, Berkeley Wellness Letter* (May 1986), P.O. Box 10922, Des Moines, Iowa 50340, © Health Letter Associates, 1986.

FIGURING THE FAT*

A simple guideline for the Maximum Metabolism Diet is that you should avoid any food that is more than 25 percent fat. But how do you figure this out? If the item is a packaged food, it's relatively easy. Here's an interpretation of a granola cereal label.

GRANOLA
CEREAL
ALL NATURAL

NUTRITION INFORMATION

SERVING SIZE	1 ounce
SERVINGS PER PACKAGE	16

Calories	130
Protein	3g
Carbohydrates	16g
Fat	6g
Sodium	95mg

PERCENTAGE OF U.S. RDA

Protein	4
Vitamin A	*
Vitamin C	*
Thiamine	6
Riboflavin	2
Niacin	2
Calcium	2
Iron	4

* Contains less than 2% U.S. RDA of this nutrient.

INGREDIENTS: Rolled oats, brown sugar, corn syrup, sugar, raisins, peanuts, honey, nonfat dry milk, salt, vegetable oil (one or more of the following: soybean, hydrogenated palm, and/or coconut oil), artificial and natural flavors, perservative BHT, MSG.

To figure out what percentage of calories comes from fat, multiply the grams of fat as listed on the label (usually under the heading "Nutrition Information") by 9 (the number of calories in 1 gram of fat) and divide this figure by the total number of calories per serving. A serving of this granola gets 42 percent of its calories from fat: 6 times 9 equals 54 fat calories, divided by 130 total calories equals .42 or 42 percent. That's a lot, since most cereals are low in fat.

*Reprinted by permission of: *University of California, Berkeley Wellness Letter*, P.O. Box 10922, Des Moines, Iowa 50340, © Health Letter Associates, 1986.

GOAL 2: Starch Only in the Morning

You need to eat just enough starch to cut down on starch cravings. But you can't have too much or you'll slow down your metabolism. You'll soon see that you are going to have to cut down on sugar completely because it is actually an addiction. But starch has a different biochemical effect on the body, so the small amount you'll be having in the morning won't be harmful.

If, after a few days on the diet, you have a truly distracting problem with starch cravings—which would probably occur in the afternoon—you can have a rice or wheat cake at that time with your fruit snack.

The typical Maximum Metabolism breakfast is cereal with skim milk and fruit. I recommend oat bran, which has been shown to stabilize blood-sugar levels and lower cholesterol. Of course, there are a number of variations on this breakfast (see pages 128–135). You can also be unorthodox and substitute a baked potato as your morning starch, as long as you don't use butter or sour cream on it. Just be sure that you relegate the starches to the morning and eliminate them from the rest of your diet.

Here are some starches you can have in the morning:

breads (½ bagel; 1 small whole-wheat pita pocket; whole wheat and other whole-grain breads; 2 slices low-calorie bread)
brown rice (½ cup cooked)
bulghur (cracked wheat)
cold cereals (Nutri-Grain, Shredded Wheat)
kasha
millet (½ cup cooked)

oat bran (raw or cooked)
oatmeal
4 rice or wheat cakes (for carbohydrate-craver morning snacks)
wheat bran
whole-grain hot cereals (Cream of Wheat, farina, etc.)
whole-grain pasta

GOAL 3: Fighting Fat with Biochemical Boosters

When I talked about cravings and hunger I mentioned the supplements that you may be using while on the Maximum Metabolism Diet. Now is the time to begin taking them. These supplements are not drugs; they are natural substances and are totally safe to take in the recommended doses. You'll find that they are an enormous help in fighting hunger and cravings as well as in controlling stress. Because you're going to be cutting down on caffeine and eliminating sugar, these biochemical boosters are particularly important because they'll give you the help you need to achieve your goals.

Please go back to Chapter 4 on Maximum Metabolism: How to Stick with It to determine which supplements you should be taking. In summary:

- Guar gum is helpful for hunger and stabilizing blood sugar. It's available in capsule form or as a powder. You should take two to four 500-milligram capsules three or four times a day before meals. Some of my patients take it between meals if they're particularly hungry.

- Chromium helps prevent sweet cravings and fatigue. It should be taken in trivalent form, which is available in a powder in a capsule. It should be taken in doses of 100 micrograms, three times a day before meals.

- Tryptophan will help you with carbohydrate cravings. Take L-tryptophan in doses of 125 milligrams between meals. You can take it with your fruit snack.

- An antistress formula vitamin will help you lose weight because, as you'll recall, stress slows your metabolism. You should begin taking your antistress formula vitamin this week. Here's the basic antistress formula that I recommend: a good-quality multiple vitamin and mineral compound containing 10,000 IUs of beta-carotene and approximately 50 milligrams of each of the B vitamins plus 1,000 milligrams of

Vitamin C, 400 IUs of Vitamin E and 50 micrograms of selenium.

In addition to the supplements you'll be taking to help fight cravings and hunger, there's another supplement you'll need to make the Maximum Metabolism Diet nutritionally complete. A diet low in fat will inevitably be low in calcium, so I recommend you take 1200 milligrams of calcium daily. Calcium is best absorbed when taken before bed.

GOAL 4: Cutting Down on Caffeine

An important goal of the Maximum Metabolism Diet is to reduce the caffeine in your diet. You will find it very difficult to succeed on this diet if you don't cut down on caffeine. In fact, I believe that unlimited caffeine can sabotage any diet.

On the Maximum Metabolism Diet you are allowed one cup of coffee, tea or decaffeinated coffee or tea per day. (Remember that decaffeinated coffee and tea still have some caffeine in them.)

I've learned from experience that I need to be emphatic about caffeine and its dangers because most of my patients don't believe me the first time around. They think they can get away with a few cups of coffee a day without any ill effects. After all, so many diets allow unlimited caffeinated beverages. In fact, some patients have come to believe that caffeine is just the boost they need to diet successfully.

Judy was such a patient. After two weeks of mixed success on the Maximum Metabolism Diet, she left me mystified. She just wasn't losing the weight that I'd anticipated. She also told me that she was hungry and had cravings, especially in the afternoon. I was beginning to think that she might be the exception that proved the rule. And then, finally, she told me she had a confession to make. She was having four cups of coffee a day. And on some days, she continued sheepishly, she'd have more.

Judy was convinced that rather than hurting her, the coffee was the key that was helping her to stick to the diet. It was true that she had headaches and cravings, and in fact if she were to be really honest she would have to admit that on a few occasions she had given in to those cravings. But she thought she was doing better than she ever had before on a diet. She was even starting to think that she ought to have more coffee when she felt afternoon cravings!

I was almost glad that Judy had spent two weeks as a caffeine cheat. It helped her to see what a difference it made when she did cut down on caffeine finally. Within two days she noticed an enormous improvement in her general energy level and the total absence of headaches and cravings. Her own body had convinced her when I couldn't.

Judy was a typical victim of the "unlimited black coffee or tea" myth that sabotages many diets. Many people have been on diets that allow them unlimited amounts of coffee or tea. Of course it must be black, or worse yet, with an artificial sweetener. The implication is that it's the cream and sugar that do the damage. This is yet another example of how the old-fashioned notion that only calories count is misleading and it is the cause of countless failed diets. In fact, I believe that unlimited caffeine is one of the most common diet breakers.

Most people don't realize that caffeine really is addictive. The Department of Health lists it along with nicotine and heroin as an addictive substance. It also goes on to say that if it were a new drug it probably would be available only by prescription.

Even more troubling than its addictive nature, from a dieter's point of view, is the fact that caffeine makes you hungry. Here's the scenario: It's 10 in the morning and you're starving. You had a light breakfast—maybe something sweet—and a cup of coffee, but now you have a slight headache and all you can think about is eating a doughnut or even a candy bar. But you're going to be good. You'll stick with a cup of coffee. So you have your coffee and you feel better immediately. Your hunger is gone and you've got that burst of energy you need to get you through the next few hours. Thank goodness for the coffee machine. But by lunchtime you're starving again and that darn headache is back. So you have a bit more lunch than you'd planned and, what the heck, that dessert. You deserve it. You're exhausted and you skipped a snack this morning. You have two cups of coffee after lunch and feel like you're ready for anything. Unfortunately, by mid-afternoon, you're exhausted again and the headache has kicked in for good.

And so it goes, day after day. You're constantly fighting a headache, you're often fighting overpowering cravings and your energy levels are wildly erratic. How could you possibly stick to a diet?

Caffeine is also a real stress on the body—one that has a negative effect on your metabolism. Remember the anti-stress hormones? They are the substances that prepare your body for an appropriate reaction to stress. Caffeine causes the release of these antistress hormones. Why does that matter to a diet? Because eventually the body's supply of these hormones is depleted. When that happens you begin to notice symptoms: fatigue, headaches, irritability and a general run-down feeling. What you aren't noticing is that due to the depletion of the antistress hormones, your metabolism is slowing down and your ability to burn calories has been compromised. You simply can't lose weight effectively, even on the best diet.

Caffeine Countdown: Identifying the Sources of Caffeine in Your Diet*

Product	Milligrams
Coffee (5-oz. cup)	
Brewed, drip method	115
Brewed, percolator	80
Instant	65
Decaffeinated, brewed	3
Decaffeinated, instant	2
Tea (5-oz. cup)	
Brewed, major U.S. brands	40
Brewed, imported brands	60
Instant	30
Iced (12-oz. glass)	70
Cocoa beverage (5-oz. cup)	4
Chocolate milk beverage (8 oz.)	5
Milk chocolate (1 oz.)	6
Dark chocolate, semisweet (1 oz.)	20
Baker's chocolate (1 oz.)	26
Chocolate-flavored syrup (1 oz.)	4
Soft Drinks (12-oz. serving)	
Mountain Dew	54.0
Mellow Yello	52.8
TAB	46.8
Coca-Cola	45.6
Diet Coke	45.6
Shasta Cola	44.4
Shasta Cherry Cola	44.4
Shasta Diet Cola	44.4
Mr. PIBB	40.8
Sugar-free Mr. PIBB	58.8
Dr Pepper	39.6
Sugar-free Dr Pepper	39.6

Product	Milligrams
Big Red	38.4
Sugar-free Big Red	38.4
Pepsi-Cola	38.4
Diet Pepsi	36.0
Pepsi Light	36.0
RC Cola	36.0
Diet Rite	36.0
Aspen	36.0
Kick	31.2
Canada Dry Jamaica Cola	30.0
Canada Dry Diet Cola	1.2

DRUGS

Prescription Drugs

Cafergot (migraine)	100
Fiorinal (tension headache)	40
Darvon Compound (pain relief)	32.4

NONPRESCRIPTION DRUGS

Weight-control aids

Codexin	200
Dex-A-Diet II	200
Dexatrim, Dexatrim Extra Strength	200
Dietac Capsules	200
Maximum Strength Appedrine	100
Prolamine	140

ALERTNESS TABLETS

Nodoz	100
Vivarin	200

ANALGESICS/PAIN RELIEVERS

Anacin, Maximum Strength Anacin	32
Excedrin	65
Midol	32.4
Vanquish	33

Product	Milligrams
DIURETICS	
Aqua-Ban	100
Maximum Strength Aqua-Ban Plus	200
Permathene H2 Off	200
COLD/ALLERGY REMEDIES	
Coryban-D capsules	30
Triaminicin tablets	30
Dristan Decongestant, Dristan	
A-F Decongestant tablets	16.2
Duradyne-Forte tablets	30
Total Daily Caffeine = _____	

* Source: National Center for Drugs and Biologics, Food and Drug Administration, March 1984

I used to ask my patients to eliminate caffeine entirely. Some did, but many simply pretended to. I've now seen that a daily cup of coffee (or tea or decaffeinated coffee), which most people prefer to have in the morning, is acceptable if that is the *only* caffeinated beverage you drink all day. Most people say, "If only I can have my morning coffee I'll be OK." And they are. But you must be sure that you don't backslide and begin to have an after-lunch cup and so on, because before you know it, you'll stop losing weight and/or you'll find it impossible to stick to the diet.

What do you drink instead? Most of my patients rely on herbal teas if they want a hot drink after their first morning cup of coffee or tea. Be sure the herbal tea you choose is caffeine-free; one widely available herbal "morning" tea has *twice* the caffeine of a cup of coffee! Remember that herbs can act as drugs; don't drink too much of any one kind. And be sure you buy herbal tea from a reliable source: People who have tried to brew their own from herbs or flowers have occasionally experienced troubling symptoms.

Most of my patients have developed a fine appreciation for seltzer and club soda, which they drink frequently either straight or with a slice of lemon or lime. At the start of dieting, most anticipate that living without regular jolts of caffeine will be difficult but they are pleasantly surprised to find that not only do they function well without caffeine overload, they actually function better than before. And, of course, the weight loss they experience is its own reward.

GOAL 5: Saying Goodbye to Sugar

Sugar is a major diet breaker and you've got to eliminate it. You must completely forgo the following:

artificial sweeteners	ice cream
cake and cookies[1]	jams and jellies[2]
candy	ketchup
chocolate	molasses
dried fruit	soda and diet soda
frozen yogurt	sugar[3]
Frozfruit bars	syrup
honey	tofutti

[1] Including sweetened health-food-store cookies.
[2] Including "naturally sweetened" types.
[3] Including brown sugar, raw sugar, turbinado sugar.

Much to your surprise, sugar can take as much of a toll on your system as caffeine. Most people think that it's only the calories in sugar that are to be avoided. In fact, that's only a small part of the picture.

When you eat too much sugar your blood-sugar levels rise to alarming heights. In response the body secretes insulin from the pancreas to escort the sugar into the cells of the body. If you're not a sugar addict, your pancreas can readily handle occasional doses of sugar. But many of us have become sugar addicts. When we eat a candy bar—which contains more sugar than your body can use in a week—your blood-sugar level goes up and your pancreas over-reacts, producing an excess of insulin. This flood of insulin depresses your blood sugar severely. In response the adrenal glands release antistress hormones, which in turn release the sugar that is stored in the liver for emergencies. The ultimate result? You feel as if you're a yo-yo: You get a brief burst of energy from the candy. Then your insulin level goes up and your spirits fall. Suddenly you feel tired, irritable, moody, depressed—and you don't know why. But finally your adrenal gland kicks in and you experience feelings of anxiety, including nervousness and sometimes even palpitations.

It all sounds pretty devastating, doesn't it? And, worst of all for a dieter, the extreme rise and fall of insulin levels makes you hungry! So sugar is making you walk a tightrope. It's causing these symptoms of energy followed by depression followed by anxiety and a constant feeling of hunger. Could you think of a worse state of mind for a dieter who's trying to stick to a sensible eating program?

In order to eliminate the sugars from your diet, you need to know where they are. It's relatively easy to eliminate table sugar but you have to be on the lookout for the secret sugars that are added to so many foods. You must read labels!

HOW MUCH SUGAR IS IN YOUR BREAKFAST CEREAL?*

You have to look very carefully to discover how much sugar there is in your cereal. Check your favorite brand; you may be surprised. For example, here's an interpretation of the label on a box of granola cereal.

GRANOLA CEREAL
ALL NATURAL

NUTRITION INFORMATION

SERVING SIZE	1 OUNCE
SERVINGS PER PACKAGE	16
Calories	130
Protein	3g
Carbohydrates	16g
Fat	6g
Sodium	95mg

PERCENTAGE OF U.S. RDA

Protein	4
Vitamin A	*
Vitamin C	*
Thiamine	6
Riboflavin	2
Niacin	2
Calcium	2
Iron	4

*Contains less than 2% U.S. RDA of this nutrient.

INGREDIENTS: Rolled oats, brown sugar, corn syrup, sugar, raisins, peanuts, honey, nonfat dry milk, salt, vegetable oil (one or more of the following: soybean, hydrogenated palm, and/or coconut oil), artificial and natural flavors, perservative BHT, MSG.

Sugars, fiber, and complex carbohydrates are lumped together under carbohydrates. A separate fiber listing is optional; it must be listed if a claim is made about it. There are no regulations concerning fiber labeling. Consumer groups have asked the FDA to make dietary fiber a mandatory part of standard labeling.

"Sugar" means sucrose (table sugar) on a label. But sugar comes in many forms, and these are listed separately, like the brown sugar, corn syrup, and honey seen here. When these are added up, sugar may actually be the predominant ingredient.

*Reprinted by permission of: *University of California, Berkeley Wellness Letter*, P.O. Box 10922, Des Moines, Iowa 50340, © Health Letter Associates, 1986.

Here are the most common sugar additives found in food:

corn syrup	mannitol
dextrose	maple syrup
fructose	molasses
glucose	sorbitol
lactose	sorghum
maltose	sucrose

When you read labels carefully, you'll be amazed to see that sugar is in everything from peanut butter to ketchup.

Though you probably won't be able to eliminate every single bit of sugar from your diet, I want you to concentrate this week on eliminating as much as you possibly can. Obviously you won't be having any candy or cake or ice cream. But I also want you to try to eliminate other, less obvious sources of sugar, such as that in spaghetti sauces and mayonnaise. Again, this is not only for the sake of reducing your intake of calories. It's for two more important reasons: First, I want to help you eliminate the sugar highs and lows and insulin rushes that will make it difficult if not impossible for you to achieve Maximum Metabolism. Second, why consume excess sugar when you don't have to? I want you to get used to reading labels and buying products that don't have sugar, whether you're officially dieting or not. For example, you can buy canned fruits, spaghetti sauces and fruit juices without sugar—there are national brands of all these items that don't contain sugar.

One of my patients told me that when she began the Maximum Metabolism Diet she occasionally ate a popular bread (I call it "foam" bread because that's what it looks and tastes like) until she read the label. When she discovered it contained corn syrup and other chemicals, she switched to bread from her local health food store. She says it really makes a difference in how she feels. In fact, her story inspired another patient to begin baking his own bread at home!

GOAL 6: Regular Meals at Regular Times

I want you to begin eating regular meals at regular times. This means that you should be having three meals a day at about the same time each day. Therefore you *must* have breakfast. Even if it's just a bowl of cereal or toast and fruit. You don't have to make a big deal of it. But you do have to have something before you begin your work day. The same with lunch. You must have a real lunch. That means 3 to 4 ounces of protein (either fish or chicken) or a salad or soup— or some other combination of foods that qualify as a proper lunch. And you must eat a real meal for dinner.

Does it sound odd to tell you to eat "real" meals? You'd be amazed at how many of my patients don't! They have nothing for breakfast, or only a doughnut and coffee at ten in the morning. Or they have just some crackers and cheese at lunch. Or they eat a huge restaurant lunch and skip both breakfast and dinner. Or they eat nothing until dinner, when it's no holds barred.

Why does this irregular eating pattern matter? Because it puts your insulin levels on a roller coaster, making it much more difficult to avoid quick fixes of sugar and caffeine and making you extremely vulnerable to cravings and binges.

Regular meals make it easier to improve your metabolism and therefore lose weight. Gordon Ball, a behavioral therapist, studied rats and their eating patterns and found that what mattered as far as weight gain was concerned was not how much was eaten at a given meal but how long the interval was between meals. The longer the interval between meals, the greater amount consumed at the next meal. If a rat ate his whole day's ration at one time, his stomach and intestines expanded, he absorbed his food 40 percent faster and he became fatter, calorie for calorie, than a rat who ate regular meals of regular size. It seems this same pattern holds true for people.

You'll be pleased to see how regular meals at regular times makes dieting easier. Michael, a securities analyst, told me: "I never realized how bad my eating habits were until I tried to eat regular meals. Most of all, I never realized how those bad eating habits were making me feel terrible as well as making me gain weight. I had gained twenty-three pounds in two years and I really think most of that weight was not because of any major pigging out on junk food but because I just ate weird things at weird times. Changing those habits made me believe I could stick to a diet, but the most important thing was that I realized how good I felt when I ate 'real' meals."

GOAL 7: Getting Active

You must start exercising! If that seems intimidating, I want you to stop thinking in terms of an exercise "program." Think simply about getting active.

If the prospect of starting an exercise program immediately seems truly impossible, then wait until you've completed two or three weeks on the Maximum Metabolism Diet.

I used to insist that patients begin to exercise immediately. I'm devoted to exercise myself and I know that its benefits are absolutely tremendous, but I now realize that postponing exercise until the benefits of your new eating pattern kick in makes far more sense than attempting a second change in your life that may be too difficult for you to deal with at the same time. Generally, you should begin an exercise program by the second week of the Maximum Metabolism Diet. People who are particularly overweight or out of shape may want to wait until the third week of the diet.

Marci told me that when she was fifty pounds overweight she couldn't face exercise. She lumped exercise and dieting together and decided that she could succeed at neither. But

"After three weeks on the diet I could see that I was really losing weight. My clothes were loose and I could hold my stomach in for the first time in ages. I surprised myself by feeling eager to exercise. I started slow and now I exercise regularly. I'm not a fanatic, but two months ago I wouldn't have believed that I'd ever be working up a sweat and enjoying it three times a week."

Remember that the benefits of exercise are absolutely *enormous* and are crucial to the success of your Maximum Metabolism program. If you add exercise to your life I promise that you will succeed in your weight-loss goal. And I promise that you'll feel better than you've felt in years, perhaps in your whole life. Get going!

My exercise suggestions are simple: If you already have some kind of exercise program—say you belong to a gym or engage in a sport at least three times a week—stick with it. But if, like most of my patients (and most people in America), you are virtually sedentary, you *must* exercise to boost your metabolism. (As I mentioned earlier, swimming is not an effective metabolism-boosting exercise.)

I've found that the three most popular and effective exercises for those who have never exercised regularly are walking, using a stationary bicycle or using an aerobic exercise video tape. Everyone can do them. They can be worked into your schedule. They can be made fun. They're simple. They're independent. Many of my patients who have never been able to stick to an exercise program have found that either walking or the stationary bicycle has been a major breakthrough for them. Some patients have adopted both: When the weather is good, they walk; in bad weather, they cycle.

Right now—today—choose the exercise you want to adopt even though you won't start until next week. It's got to be something you'll enjoy. You'll never follow through with something you don't really like.

Make sure you have comfortable clothes, including appropriate shoes if you're walking. Get any other supplies you might need. I've been amazed at the number of my patients who own an exercise bicycle that they're using as a clothes rack. Dust it off and begin slowly! If you don't own one you could probably borrow one easily if you ask around. And if you find you really enjoy it, you might want to buy your own.

If you decide to use an exercise video, be sure you get one appropriate to your level of fitness; if you begin with a very difficult one and you're a beginner, you'll become discouraged and you could also injure yourself.

Here are some suggestions for effective exercise:

- *Schedule your exercise.* This is absolutely crucial. If you decide that you'll exercise "when you have time," you never will. There will always be an excuse to avoid it. If you're using a video tape, put it on the minute you get up or just after you get in the door after work. Or whenever it's convenient for you. Many patients have told me that it's crucial to do it at the same time each day; that way it can't be put off. If you're cycling, put dinner in the oven, set the timer and ride away. Or cycle every day while you watch the morning or evening news. Or even during your favorite soap: One patient told me that cycling is the best excuse she's ever had for taking the time out for *One Life to Live.* You can even read while cycling if you invest in an inexpensive attachable bookrack.

- *Exercise at least every other day.* If you exercise less often than that, your body will not reap the metabolism-boosting benefits of exercise. Once you're a week or two into the Maximum Metabolism program you'll probably find that you *want* to exercise every day. Most of my patients report that daily exercise becomes important to them. If you haven't exercised in a long time, this may sound farfetched but, believe me, it's true.

• *Exercise at least thirty minutes at each session.* You may find that you want to extend your exercise time as you progress, but you should schedule at least a half hour for each session at the beginning. This will guarantee that you are getting an effective aerobic workout.

• *Exercise hard enough to make a difference.* The metabolism-boosting effects of exercise are felt most powerfully when your program is geared to aerobic fitness. How do you know you're exercising hard enough? First take your resting heart rate (by taking your pulse on your wrist for exactly 6 seconds and multiplying that number by 10 to get your heart rate per minute). Then use the following formula to get your target heart rate:

220 minus your age (_____) = (your maximum heart rate)
Your maximum heart rate (_____) multiplied first by .7 = your
   minimum target heart rate (_____)
Your maximum heart rate (_____) multiplied first by .85 = your
   maximum target heart rate (_____)

For example, if you are thirty-six years old, your maximum heart rate is 220 minus 36, or 184. The number 184 multiplied by .7 and .85 equals 128 and 156. Therefore, 128 to 156 is the range of your target heart rate. Your heart rate should be in that range during your exercise. If it's higher, you're working too hard; lower, not hard enough.

• *Exercise realistically.* I've found that this is the most important advice I ever give concerning exercise. Too many of my patients had given up on exercise in the past because they weren't realistic about their goals. Martin, for example, told me when he came to see me that he would follow any diet I gave him but he simply would not exercise. "I've been trying to lose weight—now I'm sixty pounds over my ideal weight—for six years. I've been on and off about ten diets and my exercise history is even worse. At least I could stick to a diet long enough to lose a few pounds, but I've never been able to exercise for more than a week. I've joined three different gyms; I never went to any of them more than four times because they really weren't convenient to either my home or my office. I bought two exercise tapes that were too difficult to follow. I tried running for four days but hurt my knee. And my wife will never let me forget that I bought a rowing machine that I just can't bring myself to use."

Martin is not unusual. There is something in us that drives us to an all-or-nothing attitude when it comes to exercise. By insisting that my patients start slowly, I've had only two exercise dropouts on the Maximum Metabolism program. Decide right now to spend your very first "exercise" session thinking about *when* and *how* and *where* you're going to exercise. Make a simple plan and stick to it.

Chapter 6

THE MAXIMUM
METABOLISM DIET PLAN

TIME AND AGAIN my patients have told me that they hate complicated diets. They're simply too busy to follow a diet that won't fit their busy lifestyles. At the same time, they need ideas for meals that taste good, are simple and conform to the principles of the Maximum Metabolism Diet.

One thing became obvious very quickly in the course of my dieting workshops: A successful diet must be flexible. Most diets are quite rigid and don't take into account the fact that some people will feel comfortable following them to the letter while others will want to pick and choose. Maximum Metabolism takes into account your personal "diet style" and makes it very easy for you to use the principles that guarantee quick and permanent weight loss.

I've found that there are three types of dieters. The Do-It-Yourself dieters want a broad outline of what they should eat and what they should avoid. They can take it from there. If this describes you and you feel comfortable devising your own Maximum Metabolism Diet plan, you can do so. You need only follow the principles in Chapter 5 on the Maximum Metabolism Basics. Use the Do's and Don'ts lists in this chapter as handy summaries of what you need to keep in mind. Then use the Maximum Metabolism Food Lists on pages 101–105 as a guide for what you can and can't eat. You'll probably want to read through the menu plans on page 91 for ideas but then you can create your own daily menus.

The Do-It-for-Me dieters want a day-by-day plan so they don't have to think. They feel comfortable knowing exactly what to shop for and what to eat every day. They're certain they're following the diet correctly because there's no guesswork. If you feel most comfortable dieting like this, follow the 21-Day Diet Plan that begins on page 106. It will give you a sequence of meals that are delicious, well-balanced and guaranteed to take advantage of every Maximum Metabolism principle. The 21-Day Diet Plan also simplifies your life by making use of dinner leftovers in many of the lunches. Of course, you can switch meals within the 21-Day Diet Plan with no ill effects: Day 3's dinner may be eaten on Day 7, for example, or any lunch may be switched with a dinner.

Most dieters are probably a combination of these types. They pick and choose. They follow some daily menus precisely. Other times, they wing it. They vary things by having the lunch at dinner and vice versa. Or they may have the same breakfast every day for two weeks. They may even have the same lunch almost every weekday. The Maximum Metabolism Diet is geared for this type of dieter too. The only principle you must watch carefully if you are a "pick-and-choose" is to confine your starches to breakfast. You can switch your lunch to dinner but you can't have your breakfast at any other time of day. Use the Do's and Don'ts lists as a handy reference and refer to the Maximum Metabolism Food Lists for inspiration.

Here's a typical day on the Maximum Metabolism Diet:

Breakfast (about 300 calories)

¾ cup hot or cold cereal
½ cup skim milk
½ cup sliced fruit

Morning Snack

1 apple or other allowed fruit

Lunch (about 300 calories)

3 to 4 ounces of protein in the form of fish or chicken, e.g.
   individual can (3½ oz.) of tuna
vegetable or greens, e.g. sliced tomato or unlimited salad,
   steamed green beans or asparagus (all with Maximum
   Metabolism dressing if desired)

Afternoon Snack

fruit (people with carbohydrate cravings may have a rice or
   wheat cake with their fruit)

Dinner (about 300 calories)

3 to 4 ounces of protein, e.g. Grilled Indian Chicken Breast
unlimited salad and/or cooked vegetables, e.g. steamed broccoli with one of the Maximum Metabolism dressings
fruit, e.g. 1 broiled banana or fruit salad

Unlimited beverages from the unlimited beverage list (page
   104).

The Maximum Metabolism Do's

- Try to eat at regular intervals. Plan to have your meals at approximately the same times each day.

- Eat grain-based carbohydrates only in the morning: whole-grain bread or muffins, rice cakes, unsweetened cold cereals, cooked grain cereals (see page 101).

- Include raw and cooked "unlimited" vegetables (see page 103) in your meals and snacks throughout the day. Leftover steamed green beans or broccoli with lemon can be a great snack.

- Include four fresh fruits daily (see page 105). You can have them as desserts or as snacks.

- Eat two 3-ounce servings of cooked fish, seafood or skinless poultry each day (remove skin from poultry *before* cooking).

- Drink water, club soda, flavored seltzers (read seltzer labels—several companies have added sugar or high-fructose corn syrup), hot or iced herbal teas, seltzer "spritzed" with unsweetened fruit juice.

- Snack on fresh fruits and vegetables.

- Season foods with herbs, mustards, vinegars, low-fat yogurt or buttermilk dressings (see recipes in Chapter 7).

- Exercise with physical activity for thirty minutes at least three times per week (after the first week or two on the diet).

The Maximum Metabolism Don'ts

- Don't eat fat. Fat occurs naturally in some of the foods in this diet and it is permissible to use a minimum amount of oil (olive oil) or vegetable cooking spray to prepare your meals. What must be avoided are foods that derive more than 25 percent of their calories from fat (see pages 68–70).

- Don't eat sugar or sweets of any kind.

- Don't use artificial sweeteners.

- Don't exceed more than one cup of coffee, tea or decaffeinated coffee or tea per day.

- Don't drink sodas or diet sodas.

- Don't eat fried foods or cream sauces.

- Don't drink more than one serving of an alcoholic beverage every other day.

- Don't use salt. Salt will make your body retain water and will raise your blood pressure. It's an enemy of good health as well as weight loss. Many of my patients have commented that once they become used to avoiding salt, their tastes change and they never miss it. Cut out table salt entirely. Choose low-sodium canned and bottled products such as tomatoes, tomato sauces, soups, broths and bouillons.

- Don't eat late meals.

- Don't skip meals.

Maximum Metabolism Breakfasts

Most of my patients want weekday breakfasts that are quick and effortless to prepare. Hot and cold cereals with fruit are the most popular Maximum Metabolism breakfasts. I've found that most people resist variety at breakfast time. They want simplicity; in fact, many of my patients have the same breakfast nearly every day except for weekends. This is fine.

Even if your breakfast is repetitive, you should take a minute to enjoy it. Please eat sitting down! You can't chew any faster standing. Take a deep breath before you begin eating and think about the day ahead of you. Think about what you are eating and how it is making you feel energized and healthy. It will help you start the day on the right note.

You'll probably want to give a bit more time to breakfast on the weekend. Many of my patients whip up a batch of muffins or pancakes on a weekend morning and freeze extras to eat during the week. Pancakes will have a slight change of texture after freezing, but muffins taste as if they're fresh-baked even after freezing. If you have a freezer stuffed with muffins and a microwave, you can have a hot muffin with some fruit—a delicious breakfast—in about one minute!

Maximum Metabolism Lunches

Diet lunches can be a challenge. Some people must eat out; others eat at their desks. Both situations call for some planning. If you eat at home, it's easier to fix an appropriate and delicious diet meal that is quick and simple but it's more difficult to resist snacking. The simple truth is that most of my patients eat sliced turkey or tuna for lunch. But of course you have other options.

For the convenience of those who eat at home or at their desks, I've tried to incorporate poultry or fish from the previous night's dinner for many of the lunches. Even though it takes another five or ten minutes to prepare lunch at home so you can bring it to work, it does give you more control over what you're eating and a far tastier lunch. And bringing your own meal allows for much greater variety than putting yourself at the mercy of your local coffee shop or deli.

If your office has a refrigerator and/or microwave, life will be easy. If not, pack chilled poultry or fish in a wide-mouth thermos bottle and wrap greens in a damp paper towel and then in a plastic bag. A small plastic container or jar is fine for dressings.

If you must rely on your local coffee shop, luncheonette or deli you face more of a challenge than ordering in a fancy restaurant. Not only is lunchtime at these places usually a fast and furious affair for the staff, making them resistant to special requests, but you yourself may find it difficult to escape the sandwich mind-set. Here are some suggestions for a Maximum Metabolism deli lunch that obviate the need to grab a sandwich:

- Individual can of water-packed tuna or salmon on a bed of greens or with a tossed salad dressed with lemon juice and/or vinegar.

- Chef's salad made with white-meat or dark-meat turkey or chicken only. Ask them to hold the ham, cheese and the dressing. Add your own lemon juice and/or vinegar.

- Sliced white-meat or dark-meat turkey with a tossed salad dressed with lemon juice and/or vinegar.

- A plate of fresh fruit. This can be a lunch in itself or your dessert.

- An all-vegetable platter. Dress with lemon juice if you wish.

Maximum Metabolism Dinners

There are any number of challenges you face when dealing with a diet dinner. If you are eating at home, you must have both the ingredients and the energy to make an appropriate meal. If you're dining out you must know how to deal with a restaurant menu. In either case, the watchword is preparation.

If you don't prepare in advance, dinner at home could be your downfall. You know how hard it is to have the energy to cook anything some nights. You can't expect to whip up the perfect, tasty, healthful meal at a moment's notice. This isn't to say that Maximum Metabolism meals are complicated; quite the contrary. But you do have to have the ingredients already on hand.

I've included a number of fish recipes for dinner and, as I think fish is at its best when it's freshest, you should plan on stopping off at a fish store the same day you'll be making a seafood meal. Most of the rest of the Maximum Metabolism dinners rely on chicken or turkey. If you have a microwave, you can defrost a chicken breast in five minutes and be well on your way to a delicious meal.

A few of my patients make a point of preparing a large bowl of salad greens on the weekend. They do all the washing, cutting and chopping and then store the greens in damp paper towels within a large plastic bag. Salad stored this way will keep for three to five days. (Don't add tomato till the last minute, as it will make the other greens soggy.) You can use the greens as a basis for any dinner salad, or lunch too.

Many of the suggested dinners make excellent lunches the next day. In fact, you may want to cook extras of some of the dinners for just that purpose. Some of my patients cook their favorite recipes in quantity and then freeze them in small containers. That way they can have dinner on the table literally in minutes.

As I mentioned earlier, you can have one alcoholic drink every other day if you wish. Don't drink any more than this.

Maximum Metabolism Restaurant Tips

If you eat out frequently, you've never had it so good as far as dieting is concerned. Most restaurants today are finally paying attention to the health concerns of diners. They are usually happy to follow reasonable special requests; if not, they don't deserve your business.

If you are choosing the restaurant, make sure it's one that has a menu featuring some light dishes. Almost every type of restaurant will have some broiled fish or chicken dish. (Though I must admit that I've never been able to come up with a Maximum Metabolism Mexican meal—too much cheese and starch!) Many restaurants today feature vegetarian dishes too. Just be sure to stick to the vegetable selections and avoid selections that feature eggs and cheese or starches such as pasta, rice and beans.

Your main restaurant challenge is to avoid fat. (You'll want to avoid starch too, but that's easy to spot. Just be sure to skip the bread, pasta, potatoes and rice.) Ask that any broiled foods be trimmed of fat and prepared without oil or butter. And request any sauce or dressing on the side. You can always request lemon and vinegar for a salad and/or lemon for vegetables.

Remember that restaurant portions are usually more than the prescribed 3 to 4 ounces of cooked meat or fish. Eat accordingly. If you wish to begin your meal with an appetizer, consommé is an excellent choice.

These key words on a restaurant menu will help you stick to your diet:

- boiled

- broiled (ask for dry-broiled)

- grilled

- poached
- steamed

Here are some key words to preparation and cooking methods that should be avoided on the Maximum Metabolism Diet, as they involve the use of oil, cream or butter:

- creamed
- deep-fried
- fried
- hollandaise
- marinated
- sautéed (except when olive oil is used)
- scalloped
- smoked
- tempura
- teriyaki

The Maximum Metabolism Food Lists

Here are lists of various foods that you'll be choosing from while on the Maximum Metabolism Diet. You'll find these lists useful for shopping and menu planning. If you're a Do-It-Yourself dieter, these lists will be the blueprint for your personalized Maximum Metabolism Diet.

Grains (³⁄₄ cup cooked serving—breakfast only)

Brown rice
Bulghur (cracked wheat)
Farina
Kasha
Millet
Oat bran (raw or cooked)
Oatmeal
Wheat bran
Wheatena
Whole-grain hot cereals (Cream of Wheat, farina, Creamy Brown Rice)
Whole-grain pasta

Cold cereals (³⁄₄ cup serving)

Nutri-Grain
Puffed Rice
Puffed Wheat
Rice Chex
Shredded Wheat
Wheat Chex

Breads

¹⁄₂ bagel
1 small whole wheat pita pocket
2 slices whole wheat and other whole-grain breads

Protein

FISH & SEAFOOD:
Abalone
Bass
Catfish
Clams (hard)
Cod
Crab
Crayfish
Flounder
Grouper
Haddock
Halibut
Lobster
Ocean Perch
Pike
Pollack
Salmon (pink)
Scallops
Sea Bass
Shrimp
Skate
Snapper
Sole
Squid
Sturgeon
Tile Fish
Trout
Tuna (fresh)
Tuna (light, in water)
POULTRY:
Chicken
   light meat without skin
   dark meat without skin
Pheasant
   without skin
Quail
   without skin

Turkey
  light meat without skin
  dark meat without skin

Vegetables (unlimited)

Artichokes
Asparagus
Broccoli
Brussels sprouts
Cabbage
Carrots
Cauliflower
Celery
Collards
Cucumber
Eggplant
Green beans
Kale
Leeks
Lettuce
Mushrooms
Mustard greens
Onions
Peppers (green, red, yellow)
Radishes
Spinach
Squash (butternut, acorn, etc.)
Swiss chard
Tomatoes
Zucchini (green, yellow)

Dairy Products (1 cup)

Buttermilk (used in dressings)
Low-fat cottage cheese (1 cup as lunch protein)
No-fat yogurt (used in dressings)
Skim or 1% milk (½ cup in morning)

High-starch Vegetables and Beans (1 medium vegetable or ½ cup cooked beans not more than twice weekly)

Potato (baked or steamed)
Sweet potato
Yam

All types of beans (e.g. limas, black, navy, kidney)
Corn
Lentils
Peas

Beverages (unlimited)

Please note that you are encouraged to drink water. The old rule about drinking eight 12-ounce glasses is fine for most people, but if you're overweight and trying to lose, you should have an extra 12-ounce glass for every 25 excess pounds of body weight. If you skimp on water consumption, you can actually slow your weight loss by slowing your metabolism: Your body simply can't work efficiently when it's denied the water essential to the metabolic process. And, by the way, drinking water will not increase your body's water retention.

Flavored seltzers (read labels and use only unsweetened brands)
Herbal teas
Lemon and water (hot or cold)
Plain seltzer
Water (keep a jar in the refrigerator; flavor with a lemon or lime slice)

Limited: 1 cup coffee, tea or decaffeinated beverage daily; 4 ounces unsweetened fruit juice daily

Fruits (choice of 4 per day)

Apple
Banana
Cantaloupe (half)
Grapefruit
Kiwi
Mango
Nectarine
Orange
Papaya
Peach
Pear
Pineapple (1 cup)
Plum
Raspberries (1 cup)
Strawberries (1 cup)
Tangerine

Unlimited lemon and lime juice for flavorings

*The 21-Day Diet Plan**

This day-by-day diet plan is for those Do-It-for-Me dieters who feel most secure when they know exactly what to eat each day. The 21-Day Diet Plan takes you by the hand and spares you any guesswork or calculating. Of course, you can substitute one dinner for another or lunch for dinner. In any case, this will be your blueprint for guaranteed weight loss.

DAY 1

Breakfast of your choice
200–300 Calories

Lunch

300 Calories

3 ounces Sliced Turkey Breast (from deli)
Mixed Green Salad with Choice of Dressing*
Pear

Dinner

350 Calories

Red Pepper Soup*
Tarragon Mustard Chicken*
Steamed Spinach
Micro-baked Apple*

* Recipes for starred items are given on pages 136–161. For breakfasts, see pages 128–135.

DAY 2

Breakfast of your choice
200–300 Calories

Lunch

260 Calories

Chicken Salad (from Day 1) with Greens and Apple
Chunks
Curried Yogurt Dressing*

Dinner

200 Calories

Marinated Grilled Swordfish*
Grilled Tomato
Steamed Green Beans

DAY 3

Breakfast of your choice
200–300 Calories

Lunch

250 Calories

3 ounces (water-packed) Tuna
Mixed Greens with Choice of Dressing*
Pear

Dinner

370 Calories

Chunky Turkey Loaf*
Steamed Acorn Squash
Micro-baked Apple*

DAY 4

Breakfast of your choice
200–300 Calories

Lunch

300 Calories

6 ounces V8 Juice
3 ounces Sliced Chunky Turkey Loaf (from Day 3)
Mixed Vegetable Salad with Choice of Dressing*
Banana

Dinner

325 Calories

Shrimp, Broccoli and Carrot Stir-fry*
Steamed Green Beans
Kiwifruit

DAY 5

Breakfast of your choice
200–300 Calories

Lunch

225 Calories

Shrimp Salad (from Day 4)
Greens and Creamy Horseradish Dressing*
Peach

Dinner

300 Calories

Sherried Oven-baked Chicken and Vegetables*
Mixed Green Salad with Dressing*
Broiled Banana

DAY 6

Breakfast of your choice
200–300 Calories

Lunch

250 Calories

Sliced Chicken (from Day 5)
Sliced Tomato with Creamy Basil Dressing*
Melon Wedge

Dinner

200 Calories

Broiled Grapefruit Half
(sprinkle with 1 tablespoon sherry if desired)
Flounder in Parchment*
Steamed Broccoli

DAY 7

Breakfast of your choice
200–300 Calories

Lunch

250 Calories

3 ounces Crabmeat on Greens with Yogurt-Dill Dressing*
1 cup strawberries

Dinner

350 Calories

Turkey Chili*
Mixed Green Salad with Dressing*
Orange

DAY 8

Breakfast of your choice
200–300 Calories

Lunch

200 Calories

Garden Minestrone Soup*
Apple

Dinner

200 Calories

Broiled Flounder with Yogurt-Dill Dressing*
Steamed Carrots
Green Salad with Lemon Juice
Melon Wedge

DAY 9

Breakfast of your choice
200–300 Calories

Lunch

200 Calories

3 ounces Sliced Turkey on Bed of Spinach with Sesame-Garlic Dressing*
Kiwifruit

Dinner

200 Calories

Broiled Bluefish with Lemon Pepper
Steamed Carrot Slices with Yogurt-Dill Dressing*

DAY 10

Breakfast of your choice
200–300 Calories

Lunch

225 Calories

3 ounces (water-packed) Tuna with Greens with Curried
Yogurt Dressing*
Apple

Dinner

250 Calories

Scallop, Snow Pea and Mushroom Stir-fry*
Mixed Green Salad with Choice of Dressing*
Tangerine

DAY 11

Breakfast of your choice
200–300 Calories

Lunch

250 Calories

3 to 4 ounces Crabmeat with Greens
2 tablespoons Lemon Dijon Dressing*
Tangerine

Dinner

300 Calories

Grilled Indian Chicken Breast*
Steamed Broccoli
Broiled Banana*

DAY 12

Breakfast of your choice
200–300 Calories

Lunch

300 Calories

Grilled Indian Chicken Salad (from Day 11)
with Greens with Yogurt-Dill Dressing*
Apple

Dinner

300 Calories

Grilled Salmon with Creamy Horseradish Dressing*
Broiled Tomato
Sliced Cucumbers
½ cup berries

DAY 13

Breakfast of your choice
200–300 Calories

Lunch

250 Calories

Salmon (from Day 12) with Greens
Sliced Cucumbers and Tomato
Nectarine

Dinner

250 Calories

Louisiana Shrimp Boil†
Steamed Asparagus with Lemon
Tomato Slices
Melon Wedge

† Available in supermarkets and seafood stores; prepare as directed.

DAY 14

Breakfast of your choice
200–300 Calories

Lunch

250 Calories

Minted Lettuce and Pea Soup*
Shrimp (from Day 13)
Tomato, Red Onion and Pepper Salad with Lemon

Dinner

320 Calories

Chicken, Broccoli and Carrot Stir-fry*
Fruit Salad

DAY 15

Breakfast of your choice
200–300 Calories

Lunch

270 Calories

Tomato (or Bell Pepper) Stuffed with Tuna Slaw*
Banana

Dinner

350 Calories

Turkey Burger*
Lettuce and Tomato Salad with Creamy Horseradish
Dressing*
Micro-baked Apple*

DAY 16

Breakfast of your choice
200–300 Calories

Lunch

200 Calories

Salad of Tuna, Tomato and Green Pepper Chunks with
Curried Yogurt Dressing* on Greens
Kiwifruit

Dinner

300 Calories

Chili-Rubbed Chicken*
½ cup Cooked Black Beans
Mixed Green Salad with Choice of Dressing*
Tomato Slices with Lime Juice

DAY 17

Breakfast of your choice
200–300 Calories

Lunch

200 Calories

Salad of Diced Turkey, Tomato and Pepper Chunks with Choice of Dressing*
Orange

Dinner

275 Calories

Mediterranean Fish Stew*
Melon Wedge

DAY 18

Breakfast of your choice
200–300 Calories

Lunch

200 Calories

Tuna on Greens with Dressing*
6 ounces Tomato Juice

Dinner

300 Calories

Grilled or Broiled Turkey Breast (4 ounces)
(grill 4 ounces extra for lunch on Day 19)
Arugula, Tomato and Red Onion Salad with Choice of
Dressing*
Pear

DAY 19

Breakfast of your choice
200–300 Calories

Lunch

200 Calories

4 ounces Sliced Turkey Breast (from Day 18)
on Greens with Tomato Chunks
Creamy Horseradish Dressing*

Dinner

250 Calories

Broiled Bluefish with Dijon Dill Glaze*
Steamed Green Beans and Carrots
Mango Half

DAY 20

Breakfast of your choice
200–300 Calories

Lunch

225 Calories

Cold Bluefish (from Day 19) on Greens with Yogurt-Dill
Dressing*
Pear

Dinner

200 Calories

Shrimp Scampi*
(microwave 3 ounces extra for 3 minutes for lunch on
Day 21)
Steamed Broccoli
Melon Wedge

DAY 21

Breakfast of your choice
200–300 Calories

Lunch

250 Calories

Shrimp Cocktail (from Day 20)
on Greens
2 tablespoons Cocktail Sauce
Banana

Dinner

325 Calories

Chicken Mushroom Sauté*
Steamed Cauliflower and Carrots
Micro-baked Apple*

Chapter 7

THE MAXIMUM METABOLISM RECIPES

H ERE ARE RECIPES for the starred items in the 21-Day Diet Plan as well as some breakfast recipes. Many of the recipes have been suggested by my patients, who have been extremely creative in coming up with dishes that are consistent with the Maximum Metabolism goals. In fact, I think of them as "real recipes for real people" because they're very much in tune with the way ordinary people diet successfully. They're all simple—and I can promise you they're all delicious!

BREAKFAST MENUS AND RECIPES

Here are some tempting breakfast ideas to start your day on The Maximum Metabolism Diet.

Diet Classic Breakfast

About 300 Calories

Deciphering ingredients on cereal boxes is no easy task. There are more forms of sugar and salt than most of us imagine. Here are some good cold cereal choices: Nutri-Grain, Puffed Rice or Puffed Wheat, Oat Bran or Shredded Wheat.

3/4 cup cold cereal
1/2 cup skim milk
1/2 cup sliced fruit

Quick Comfort Breakfast

About 250 Calories

Memories of old-fashioned breakfasts of steaming oatmeal can be conjured up in seconds. Now with the microwave they can also be cooked almost as quickly—and there's no messy pan to clean.

If you are not a fan of creamy hot cereal textures, take heart: There is a deliciously chewy oatmeal called McCann's Irish Oatmeal. Its slightly nutty toasted flavor will make you an instant convert. For a variation, try shredding 1/2 cup apple into the cereal mixture before cooking.

3/4 cup cooked hot cereal
1/2 cup skim milk
1/2 banana or other fruit

Crunchy Quick Breakfast

About 300 Calories

There are some days when there is only time for toast, picked up at the local coffee shop on the way to work. This doesn't have to be the start of a bad day. Choose whole-grain bread, toasted dry, orange juice and a decaffeinated beverage. If you are eating at home, you can spread the toast with a pureed fruit such as apple butter. Take the time to savor what you are eating.

½ cup orange juice
2 slices whole-grain toast
apple butter
decaffeinated coffee or tea

Gem of a Breakfast

About 200 Calories

Double Bran Gem Muffins—some of my patients tell me that they are the best bran muffins they have ever eaten! I'm not surprised, just pleased that most of the fat in them has been replaced by pureed fruit. And chunks of strawberries and pineapple will evoke summertime even on the darkest of days.

1 cup strawberry and pineapple chunks
1 Double Bran Gem Muffin*
decaffeinated coffee or tea

Double Bran Gem Muffins

In addition to being delicious, these muffins are an excellent source of fiber: they'll satisfy your hunger as they aid your regularity.

1   cup wheat bran
1   cup oat bran
1   cup whole-wheat flour
2   teaspoons baking powder
1   teaspoon baking soda
1/2   teaspoon cinnamon
1/2   teaspoon nutmeg
2   large bananas, mashed
1/2   cup skim milk
2   egg whites, lightly beaten
2   tablespoons olive oil

Preheat oven to 400 degrees. Line a 12-cup muffin pan with paper muffin liners or spray each cup with non-stick cooking spray.

In a large bowl combine wheat and oat bran, whole-wheat flour, baking powder, baking soda, cinnamon and nutmeg. In another bowl combine mashed bananas, milk, egg whites and oil. Pour onto dry ingredients and mix until just combined. Scoop by 1/4 cupfuls into prepared muffin cups. Bake 14 to 16 minutes, or until toothpick inserted in center is sticky but not wet.

Makes 12 muffins.

Per muffin: 100 calories; 3 grams protein; 18 grams carbohydrate; 3 grams fat; 190 milligrams sodium.

Country Inn Breakfast

About 200 Calories

The aroma of Cinnamon-Orange Oat Muffins will make you forget that you are dieting. And the taste will keep you smiling. Freeze the muffins that you don't plan to eat in the next day or two—then at the desired time just pop in the microwave for 30 seconds or bake in the toaster oven at 350 degrees for 5 minutes.

1 Cinnamon-Orange Oat Muffin*
½ cup fruit
decaffeinated coffee or tea

Cinnamon-Orange Oat Muffins

The oat bran in these muffins help to stabilize your blood sugar and lower your cholesterol. You can freeze extras and reheat them in a microwave in seconds for a tempting breakfast.

1 cup rolled oats
1 cup oat bran
1 cup whole-wheat flour
2 teaspoons baking power
1 teaspoon baking soda
1 teaspoon cinnamon
1 teaspoon grated orange rind
1 cup unsweetened applesauce
¾ cup low-fat buttermilk
2 egg whites, lightly beaten
2 tablespoons olive oil

Preheat oven to 400 degrees. Line a 12-cup muffin pan with paper muffin liners or spray each cup with non-stick cooking spray.

In a large bowl combine oats, bran, flour, baking powder, baking soda and cinnamon. In another bowl beat together orange rind, applesauce, buttermilk, egg whites and oil. Pour onto dry ingredients and mix until just combined. Scoop by ¼ cupfuls into prepared muffin cups. Bake 15 to 17 minutes, or until toothpick inserted in center is sticky but not wet.

Makes 12 muffins.

Per muffin: 115 calories; 4 grams protein; 19 grams carbohydrate; 3 grams fat; 160 milligrams sodium.

Brunchy Breakfast Omelet

About 200 Calories

Green peppers and a handful of sliced mushrooms make this easy omelet deliciously healthy. This is a breakfast that will take about 10 minutes to prepare. It's worth taking the time to make it and you'll want another 10 minutes to savor the flavors.

6 ounces tomato juice
Mushroom Pepper Omelet*
1 slice whole-grain toast
decaffeinated coffee or tea

Mushroom Pepper Omelet

There's no need to feel deprived because you're changing your eating habits. This yolk-free omelet is light and flavorful. It's ideal for Sunday mornings.

½ cup green pepper, thinly sliced
½ cup mushrooms, sliced
2 egg whites
1 tablespoon water
⅛ teaspoon black pepper

Spray a small skillet with non-stick cooking spray. Add peppers and mushrooms and cook over high heat for 5 minutes, stirring occasionally. Scoop mixture onto plate. Wipe skillet, spray again with cooking spray.
Combine egg whites, water and pepper; heat until blended. Heat skillet over medium low heat. Pour egg mixture into skillet; cover and cook 2 minutes, or until set. Scoop vegetables onto one half of omelet. Fold top over.
Makes 1 serving.
60 calories; 8 grams protein; 4 grams carbohydrate; 1 gram fat; 100 milligrams sodium.

House of Pancakes Breakfast

About 200 Calories

A Sunday morning, free time to read the newspaper and make a batch of Fluffy Oat Pancakes. For an added treat make some Spiced Apple Syrup, redolent of cinnamon and cloves and a perfect match for these slightly nutty pancakes.

Freeze any extra pancakes and reheat in the microwave or pop in the toaster oven for a simple mid-week breakfast.

3 Fluffy Oat Pancakes*
2 tablespoons Spiced Apple Syrup*
decaffeinated coffee or tea

Fluffy Oat Pancakes

These pancakes are the real thing—hearty and delicious. And the syrup, which was suggested by one of my patients, has been a hit with everyone because it's so good and so easy to prepare.

1/2	cup rolled oats
1/4	cup oat bran
1/4	cup whole-wheat flour
1/2	teaspoon baking soda
1	cup low-fat buttermilk
1	teaspoon vanilla
2	egg whites

Heat electric griddle to 370 degrees or heat a heavy skillet over medium-high heat. In a large bowl combine oats, bran, flour, baking soda, buttermilk and vanilla; set aside.

In a clean mixer bowl beat egg whites until soft peaks form. Fold egg whites into oat mixture. Lightly wipe griddle or skillet with oil or non-stick cooking spray.

Scoop batter onto griddle or skillet in scant 1/4 cupfuls and cook until bubbles form on tops of pancakes. Turn pancakes and cook 1 minute more. Serve with Spiced Apple Syrup if desired.

Makes 9 pancakes (3 servings).

Per serving: 140 calories; 9 grams protein; 23 grams carbohydrate; 2 grams fat; 280 milligrams sodium.

Spiced Apple Syrup

In a small saucepan combine one 6-oz. can unsweetened apple juice concentrate, 2 whole cloves, 1 cinnamon stick and 1/4 cup water; heat to boiling. Simmer 5 minutes, or until syrup measures 3/4 cup.

Makes 6 servings.

Per serving: 40 calories; trace protein; 10 grams carbohydrate; trace fat; 6 milligrams sodium.

Dessert for Breakfast

About 300 Calories

Feeling devilish? Try cinnamon-baked apple chunks topped with a handful of Nutri-Grain cereal that's been "crunched" in the microwave. It's like having dessert for breakfast!

Breakfast Apple Crisp*
1/2 cup skim milk
decaffeinated coffee or tea

Breakfast Apple Crisp

This crisp is a real treat for breakfast. And it's a snap to prepare—even on a busy morning.

1   red or golden Delicious apple
1/4   teaspoon cinnamon
1/2   cup Nutri-Grain or other approved cereal

Cut apple into 3/4-inch chunks. Place in a microwaveproof bowl and sprinkle with cinnamon. Cover with plastic wrap and microwave on High for 3 minutes. Uncover and sprinkle with cereal. Microwave 1 minute more.

Makes 1 serving.

280 calories; 7 grams protein; 68 grams carbohydrate; 1 gram fat; 390 milligrams sodium.

SOUPS

Red Pepper Soup

The sweetness of red peppers is a perfect balance to the tangy buttermilk. The simple method used in this pureed soup works well with any full-flavored vegetable (try celery, carrot, tomato, cucumber with green onion). The most difficult decision you'll have is whether to serve it hot or chilled!

2	red peppers, cored, seeded and chopped
1½	cups water
1	low-sodium chicken bouillon cube
¼	teaspoon thyme
1	cup low-fat buttermilk
	ground black pepper

In a medium saucepan combine peppers, water, bouillon and thyme. Heat to boiling; cover and simmer over medium-low heat for 10 minutes. Cool slightly. Transfer to blender and puree until smooth. Add buttermilk and blend until combined. Return to saucepan and heat through, but do not boil or cover. Refrigerate 4 hours, or until completely chilled. Dust with freshly ground black pepper before serving.

Makes 3 servings (3 cups).

Per serving: 45 calories; 4 grams protein; 8 grams carbohydrate; 1 gram fat; 110 grams sodium.

Minted Lettuce and Pea Soup

In certain culinary circles this soup is called Potage Saint-Germain. The subtle sweetness of the mint and the peas bring to mind the bounty of a summer to come. Serve hot or chilled.

2   cups water
3   cups Boston lettuce (do not shred)
1   cup frozen peas
1   teaspoon fresh, or dried mint
1   low-sodium chicken bouillon cube
½   cup low-fat yogurt
¼   teaspoon black pepper

In a medium saucepan combine water, lettuce, frozen peas, mint and bouillon. Cover and cook over high heat 5 minutes. Cool slightly. Transfer to blender and puree until almost smooth. Add yogurt and pepper and blend until combined. Return to saucepan and heat through without boiling.

Makes 3 servings (3 cups).

Per serving: 75 calories; 5 grams protein; 12 grams carbohydrate; 1 gram fat; 75 grams sodium.

Garden Minestrone Soup

This quick version of homemade minestrone features root vegetables and broccoli. You can vary the vegetables (choose from the unlimited vegetable list on page 103) at your whim—zucchini, cauliflower, spinach, kale or snow peas are also delicious. If you have parsley or oregano on hand, add them in the last few minutes for a wonderful fresh flavor.

1	teaspoon olive oil
1/2	cup onions, sliced
1	cup carrots, sliced
1	cup celery, diced
3	cups water
1	16-oz. can whole tomatoes
1	low-sodium chicken bouillon cube
1	tablespoon chopped fresh basil (or 1/2 teaspoon dry)
1/2	teaspoon thyme
1	garlic clove, pressed
1	16-oz. can kidney beans, rinsed and drained
1	cup broccoli flowerets

In a large saucepan heat oil over medium-high heat. Add onions; cover and cook 2 minutes. Add carrots, celery, water, tomatoes, bouillon, basil, thyme and garlic, cover and heat to boiling. Uncover and simmer 10 minutes. Stir in beans and broccoli and simmer 5 minutes more.

Makes 6 servings.

Per serving: 100 calories; 5 grams protein; 17 grams carbohydrate; 1 gram fat; 320 milligrams sodium.

MAIN COURSES

Tarragon Mustard Chicken

If you live in an area where fresh tarragon is available (or are lucky enough to have an herb garden), by all means use a teaspoon of it instead of dried tarragon. Its more delicate flavor will also work well with the mustard.

- 8   ounces boned skinless chicken breasts
- ¼   teaspoon tarragon
- ¼   cup dry white wine
- 1   teaspoon Dijon mustard

Spray a medium skillet with non-stick cooking spray. Heat over medium-high heat. Add chicken breasts and cook 3 minutes; turn breasts and cook 2 minutes more. Remove and set aside. Add tarragon, white wine and mustard to skillet and cook over high heat until juices are syrupy, about 2 minutes. Pour juices over chicken. (Set aside one half of the chicken for tomorrow's lunch.)

Makes 2 servings.

Per serving: 190 calories; 30 grams protein; trace carbohydrate; 4 grams fat; 145 milligrams sodium.

Marinated Grilled Swordfish

Swordfish is always a special treat. Treated here as a steak, swordfish can also be cut into 1-inch chunks and skewered alternately with wedges of onion and pepper and grilled.

2   tablespoons lemon juice
⅛   teaspoon thyme
⅛   teaspoon black pepper
1   small garlic clove, slivered
4   ounces swordfish

On a dinner plate combine all ingredients except swordfish. Add swordfish and turn to coat both sides with marinade; let stand 10 minutes.

Preheat broiler or grill. Place swordfish on broiler rack 3 inches from heat source and broil 3 minutes. Turn and broil 1 to 2 minutes more. NOTE: Timing will vary with thickness of fish. Allow about 5 minutes per ½ inch of thickness.

Makes 1 serving.

145 calories; 22 grams protein; 4 grams carbohydrate; 5 grams fat; 2 milligrams sodium.

Chunky Turkey Loaf

This colorful vegetable-studded loaf has all the old-fashioned flavor of a traditional meat loaf without the fat. The addition of the tomato juice gives a succulent juiciness sometimes lacking in ground turkey preparations. Leftovers heat well in the microwave—you can even freeze individual cooked portions for weeks ahead. And one of my patients raves about a "short-cut" version of this made with the turkey, onion, ¼ cup chopped mushrooms and the spices.

1	pound ground turkey
¼	cup onion, chopped
¼	cup carrot, chopped
¼	cup celery, chopped
¼	cup red or green pepper, cored, seeded and chopped
1	garlic clove, pressed
¼	teaspoon thyme
¼	teaspoon nutmeg
⅛	teaspoon black pepper
¼	cup tomato juice
1	tomato, sliced

Preheat oven to 350 degrees. Spray an 8-inch-square baking dish with non-stick cooking spray or line with foil.

In a large bowl combine all ingredients and mix until just blended. Shape into a 6-inch oval loaf. Arrange tomato slices over top and bake 1 hour.

Makes 4 servings.

Per serving: 105 calories; 15 grams protein; 5 grams carbohydrate; 2 grams fat; 188 milligrams sodium.

Shrimp, Broccoli and Carrot Stir-fry

A veritable explosion of color and flavor, this simple stir-fry meal will certainly become part of your repertoire. You can play with vegetable combinations (green onion, carrot, cauliflower) or substitute chicken, turkey or fish for the shrimp.

1/2	teaspoon olive oil
1	teaspoon grated fresh ginger
1	small garlic clove, pressed
	Pinch red pepper flakes
1	large carrot, cut in 1/4-inch slices
1	cup broccoli flowerets
4	tablespoons water
4	ounces shrimp, shelled, deveined and split lengthwise
1	teaspoon low-sodium soy sauce
1/4	teaspoon sesame oil

In a wok or large skillet, heat oil over high heat. Add ginger, garlic, red pepper flakes, carrot and broccoli; stir-fry 1 minute.

Add 2 tablespoons water; cover and cook 2 minutes.

Uncover and stir in shrimp; stir-fry 2 minutes more. Stir in remaining 2 tablespoons water, soy sauce and sesame oil; heat through.

Makes 1 serving.

190 calories; 22 grams protein; 15 grams carbohydrate; 4 grams fat; 370 milligrams sodium.

Sherried Oven-baked Chicken and Vegetables

There are some dishes that can fool the palate: This simply baked combination of root vegetables enhanced with garlic, mushrooms and a splash of sherry is reminiscent of a French farmhouse preparation that takes hours longer to prepare and would add hundreds more calories to your daily tally. Bon appétit!

½	cup carrot, sliced
¼	cup onion, sliced
¼	cup celery, diced
1	whole chicken breast, split and skinned
½	cup mushrooms, sliced
1	garlic clove, pressed
¼	cup boiling water
2	tablespoons dry sherry or vermouth

Preheat oven to 400 degrees. In a small casserole, combine carrot, onion and celery. Place chicken on top, bone side down. Arrange mushrooms over chicken and sprinkle with garlic. Combine boiling water and sherry; add mixture to casserole. Cover and bake 35 minutes. Reserve one half-breast for tomorrow's lunch. Serve remaining chicken with vegetables and juices.

Makes 2 servings total.

Per serving: 171 calories; 28 grams protein; 8 grams carbohydrate; 3 grams fat; 91 milligrams sodium.

Flounder in Parchment

Cooking in parchment (en papillote) *steams the food and releases natural juices, leaving your ingredients bathed in a luscious sauce. This technique is so easy and gives such delicious results that you'll want to try it with boneless poultry as well. If parchment is not available, foil is a fine substitute.*

4	ounces flounder fillet
1	small carrot, thinly sliced
4	mushrooms, thinly sliced
1	green onion, thinly sliced
1	teaspoon chopped fresh dill (or ¼ teaspoon dried)
	Freshly ground black pepper

Preheat oven to 400 degrees. Cut a sheet of baking parchment paper or aluminum foil into an oval slightly larger than the size of a dinner plate; fold in half.

Open parchment and place fish to one side of and parallel to the centerfold. Top with remaining ingredients. Fold parchment over ingredients and fold edges at ½-inch intervals to seal. Place on a cookie sheet and bake 12 minutes. Carefully slit open with a knife to serve.

Makes 1 serving.

125 calories; 20 grams protein; 9 grams carbohydrate; 1 gram fat; 115 milligrams sodium.

Turkey Chili

The addition of green chilies to this simple dish takes it out of the realm of the ordinary. The chilies round out the flavor and add a mellowness that will please any Tex-Mex aficionado. Leftovers freeze very well—pack in individual containers and reheat in the microwave.

One of my patients passed on this tip about turkey chili: You can use a commercial chili seasoning kit (for example, Two-Alarm brand) to make a great chili. Omit the salt (which comes in a separate envelope) or use just a pinch.

1	teaspoon olive oil
½	cup onion, chopped
2	teaspoons chili powder
1	teaspoon ground cumin
1	garlic clove, pressed
1	pound ground turkey
1	16-oz. can whole tomatoes
1	4-oz. can chopped green chilies, drained

In a medium saucepan, heat oil over medium-high heat. Add onion; cover and cook 2 minutes. Stir in chili powder, cumin and garlic; cook 1 minute. Add turkey and cook 3 minutes more, until pinkness is gone. Stir in tomatoes and green chilies; cover and heat to boiling.

Makes 4 servings.

Per serving: 130 calories; 15 grams protein; 8 grams carbohydrate; 3.5 grams fat; 300 milligrams sodium.

Tomato Stuffed with Tuna Slaw

With just a few minutes of advance preparation you can make this diet staple into an elegant lunch. The Creamy Basil Dressing is especially delicious with the tuna, but any of the other permitted dressings pages will work wonders too.

1 large tomato (or bell pepper)
3 ounces water-packed low-sodium tuna
1 small rib celery, thinly sliced
1 small carrot, shredded
2 tablespoons Creamy Basil Dressing (page 157)
 Pinch black pepper

Remove core from tomato. Cut a quarter-inch slice from end; scoop out center of tomato and chop up. Transfer to a mixing bowl and add remaining ingredients until thoroughly combined. Mound tuna slaw into tomato shell.

Serves 1.

170 calories; 25 grams protein; 17 grams carbohydrate; 1 gram fat; 300 milligrams sodium.

Scallop, Snow Pea and Mushroom Stir-fry

Snowy white scallops, crunchy snow peas and the gentle warmth of fresh ginger will make this dish a favorite for a quick and elegant dinner. For an added gourmet touch, use shitake mushrooms in place of the cultivated ones.

½   teaspoon olive oil
1   teaspoon grated fresh ginger
2   green onions, cut in 1-inch pieces
2   tablespoons water
4   ounces scallops, cut in slices
½   cup mushrooms, sliced
2   ounces (about 24) snow peas
2   tablespoons water
1   teaspoon low-sodium soy sauce
¼   teaspoon sesame oil

In a wok or large skillet, heat olive oil over high heat: Add ginger and onions; stir-fry 1 minute. Add 2 tablespoons water; cover and cook 2 minutes. Add scallops and mushrooms and cook 3 minutes more. Stir in snow peas, water, soy sauce and sesame oil; cover and cook 1 minute more. Makes 1 serving.

140 calories; 16 grams protein; 9 grams carbohydrate; 4 grams fat; 350 milligrams sodium.

Grilled Indian Chicken Breast

This succulent chicken dish takes its inspiration from the Indian tradition of cooking with the tandoor, a clay oven in which marinated meats and seafoods are cooked to juicy perfection.

Marinade

- ½ cup low-fat yogurt
- 1 small onion, quartered
- ½ teaspoon ground cumin powder
- ½ teaspoon ground coriander powder
- ½ teaspoon curry powder
- 1 small peeled clove garlic, whole
- 8 ounces boned skinless chicken breasts

In blender combine all marinade ingredients; puree until smooth. Place chicken breasts in a shallow dish. Pour marinade over and turn chicken to coat. Cover and let stand at least 15 minutes. (This can be done in advance. Cover and refrigerate up to 24 hours before final cooking.)

Preheat grill or broiler or heat a large cast-iron skillet over medium-high heat. Spray cooking surface lightly with nonstick cooking spray. Cook chicken 4 minutes per side. Serve 1 breast half per serving.

Makes 2 servings.

Per serving: 190 calories; 32 grams protein; 4 grams carbohydrate; 4 grams fat; 90 milligrams sodium.

Turkey Burgers

These lean-meat variations on beefy hamburgers are a cinch to prepare. Experiment with seasonings: thyme, marjoram, allspice, etc.

4   ounces ground turkey meat
1   tablespoon chopped onion
1   tablespoon chopped green pepper
    dash of low-sodium Worcestershire sauce
1   teaspoon tomato paste

Preheat broiler. In small bowl combine all ingredients until blended. Shape into patty. Place on sheet of aluminum foil on broiler rack 3 inches from heat. Broil 3 minutes, turn and broil 3 additional minutes.

Makes 1 serving.

Per serving: 105 calories; 15 grams protein; 2 grams carbohydrate; 2 grams fat; 130 milligrams sodium.

Chicken, Broccoli and Carrot Stir-fry

This is a quick, easy meal with lots of flavor. For more zip, add a pinch of hot red pepper flakes along with the ginger and garlic.

1	teaspoon olive oil
1/2	cup carrots, sliced
1/4	cup onion, sliced
1	teaspoon grated fresh ginger
1	garlic clove, pressed
4	ounces chicken chunks
1/4	cup water
1	cup broccoli flowerets
2	tablespoons water
1	teaspoon low-sodium soy sauce
1/4	teaspoon sesame oil

In a wok or large skillet, heat oil over high heat. Stir in carrots, onion, ginger and garlic; stir-fry 1 minute. Add chicken and stir-fry 1 more minute. Pour in the 1/4 cup water; cover and cook 2 minutes. Add broccoli and remaining 2 tablespoons water; cover and cook 3 minutes more. Stir in soy sauce and sesame oil and heat through.

Makes 1 serving.

210 calories; 13.5 grams protein; 16 grams carbohydrate; 4 grams fat; 300 milligrams sodium.

Chili-Rubbed Chicken

This is one of the easiest chicken preparations ever, yet there is something indescribably satisfying about the slight heat of the chili paired with the creaminess of black beans.

4 ounces boned skinless chicken breasts
1 garlic clove, pressed
½ teaspoon chili powder

Preheat grill or broiler or heat a large cast-iron skillet over medium-high heat.

Pat chicken dry with paper towel. Rub breasts with garlic and then sprinkle with the chili powder. Cook 3 minutes; turn and cook 2 minutes more. Serve with ½ cup cooked black beans.

Makes 1 serving.

165 calories; 31 grams protein; 1 gram carbohydrate; 4 grams fat; 70 milligrams sodium.

Mediterranean Fish Stew

Each small town along the Mediterranean has its own version of a seafood stew. This full-flavored one in the Provençal tradition uses a touch of fennel and some tomato. If cod is not available, try halibut, haddock, orange roughy or pollock. You could also use squid; if you do, cut it into rings and add during the last 2 minutes of cooking.

1   teaspoon olive oil
1   garlic clove, pressed
¼   teaspoon fennel seeds
     Pinch hot red pepper flakes
1   large tomato or 3 plum tomatoes, chopped
½   cup bottled clam juice
½   cup dry white wine
4   ounces cod or other firm-fleshed fish, cut in ½-inch chunks
4   ounces shrimp, peeled, deveined and split lengthwise
8   mussels (about ¾ lb.), scrubbed

In a large saucepan, heat oil over medium heat. Stir in garlic, fennel and red pepper flakes; cook 1 minute. Add tomatoes, clam juice and wine; bring to a boil then cover and simmer 5 minutes. Increase heat to high. Add cod; cover and cook 3 minutes. Add shrimp and mussels; cover and cook 2 minutes more or until mussels open.

Makes 2 servings.

Per serving: 225 calories; 30 grams protein; 8 grams carbohydrate; 7 grams fat; 260 milligrams sodium.

Bluefish with Dijon Dill Glaze

When bluefish is fresh it can be one of the most delicate, moist fruits of the sea. The glaze is a perfect complement to its sweetness.

4   ounces bluefish fillet
1   tablespoon lemon juice
1   tablespoon low-fat yogurt
1   teaspoon Dijon mustard
1   teaspoon chopped fresh dill
    Pinch ground black pepper

Preheat broiler. Place bluefish on broiler rack 3 inches from heat source. Broil 4 minutes. Meanwhile, combine remaining ingredients in a small bowl. Spoon glaze over fish and broil 2 minutes more, or until desired doneness.

Makes 1 serving.

130 calories; 21 grams protein; 2 grams carbohydrate; 4 grams fat; 155 milligrams sodium.

Shrimp Scampi

The touch of fresh basil paired with lemon gives this meal a richness of flavor that you'll want to try on other foods. It works very nicely with chicken or turkey cutlets, for example. The scampi also make great "toothpick food" if you're hosting a party.

- ½ teaspoon olive oil
- 1 garlic clove, pressed
- 4 ounces shrimp, peeled, deveined and split lengthwise
- 1 tablespoon chopped fresh basil (or parsley)
- 2 tablespoons lemon juice
  Freshly ground black pepper

In a small skillet, heat oil over medium heat. Stir in garlic and cook until garlic begins to color. Add shrimp and cook about 3 minutes, until they curl and turn bright pink. Stir in basil and lemon juice; toss a few seconds. Season with pepper.

Makes 1 serving.

125 calories; 18 grams protein; 5 grams carbohydrate; 4 grams fat; 130 milligrams sodium.

Chicken Mushroom Sauté

Sautéeing is a versatile technique. The simple ingredients used here can be embellished with the addition of ¼ cup frozen peas (thawed), or by substituting vermouth or brandy for the white wine.

1 teaspoon olive oil

1 small garlic clove, pressed

4 ounces boned skinless chicken breasts, cut in ½-inch chunks

1 cup mushrooms, quartered

2 tablespoons white wine

¼ cup water

In a small skillet, heat oil over medium-high heat. Add garlic and chicken pieces and cook, stirring, 3 minutes. Stir in mushrooms and cook 3 minutes more. Scoop chicken and mushrooms onto serving plate. Pour wine and water into skillet and boil 1 minute over high heat. Pour juices over chicken.

Makes 1 serving.

240 calories; 32 grams protein; 5 grams carbohydrate; 8 grams fat; 75 milligrams sodium.

Dressings

Variety is the spice of life. The following recipes should give both to your diet routine. In addition to their use as salad dressings, the yogurt- and buttermilk-based dressings can also be used either cold or brushed over an almost-cooked piece of poultry or fish for the last minute or two of cooking to give a nice glaze, and of course, added flavor.

Creamy Horseradish

- ½   cup low-fat yogurt
- 2   tablespoons prepared horseradish
- ⅛   teaspoon black pepper

Combine all ingredients in a small bowl. Mix until well blended. Makes 8 tablespoons.

Per 2-tablespoon serving: 20 calories; 1 gram protein; 2 grams carbohydrate; .5 grams fat; 100 milligrams sodium.

Dijon Vinaigrette

- ½   cup red or white wine vinegar
- 1   tablespoon olive oil
- 2   tablespoons Dijon mustard
- 1   tablespoon water
- ¼   teaspoon black pepper

Combine all ingredients in a jar with a tight-fitting lid; cover and shake until well blended. Makes 10 tablespoons.

Per 2-tablespoon serving: 47 calories; trace protein; 1 gram carbohydrate; 3 grams fat; 175 milligrams sodium.

Lemon Dijon

¼ cup low-fat yogurt
2 tablespoons lemon juice
1 tablespoon Dijon mustard
½ teaspoon tarragon
⅛ teaspoon black pepper

Combine all ingredients in a small bowl. Mix until well blended. Makes 8 tablespoons.
Per 2-tablespoon serving: 15 calories; 1 gram protein; 2 grams carbohydrate; .5 grams fat; 120 milligrams sodium.

Sesame-Garlic

½ cup brown rice vinegar
2 tablespoons low-sodium soy sauce
1 teaspoon sesame oil
1 teaspoon grated fresh ginger
1 garlic clove, pressed

Combine all ingredients in a small jar with a tight-fitting lid; cover and shake until well blended. Makes 10 tablespoons.
Per 2-tablespoon serving: 15 calories; .5 grams protein; 2 grams carbohydrate; 1 gram fat; 240 milligrams sodium.

Creamy Basil

½ cup low-fat buttermilk
2 tablespoons chopped fresh basil
1 teaspoon cider vinegar
⅛ teaspoon black pepper

Combine all ingredients in a small bowl. Mix until well blended. Makes 8 tablespoons.
Per 2-tablespoon serving: 15 calories; 1 gram protein; 2 grams carbohydrate; trace fat; 40 milligrams sodium.

Spicy Tomato

³/₄ cup tomato juice
¹/₄ cup red or white wine vinegar
 1   tablespoon olive oil
¹/₄ teaspoon oregano
¹/₄ teaspoon thyme
¹/₈ teaspoon ground red pepper (cayenne)

Combine all ingredients in a jar with a tight-fitting lid; cover and shake until well blended. Makes 16 tablespoons.

Per 2-tablespoon serving: 20 calories; trace protein; 1 gram carbohydrate; 1.5 grams fat; 80 milligrams sodium.

Yogurt-Dill

 1   cup low-fat yogurt
¹/₄ cup chopped fresh dill
 1   tablespoon cider vinegar
¹/₈ teaspoon black pepper

Combine all ingredients in a small bowl. Mix until well blended. Makes 16 tablespoons.

Per 2-tablespoon serving: 20 calories; 2 grams protein; 2 grams carbohydrate; 1 gram fat; 20 milligrams sodium.

Curried Yogurt

¹/₂ cup low-fat yogurt
 1   teaspoon curry powder
 1   teaspoon lemon juice

Combine all ingredients in a small bowl. Mix until well blended. Makes 8 tablespoons.

Per 2-tablespoon serving: 10 calories; .5 grams protein; 1 gram carbohydrate; trace fat; 10 milligrams sodium.

Ketchup

1	teaspoon dry mustard
1/8	teaspoon nutmeg
1/8	teaspoon ground cloves
2	teaspoons white vinegar
1	teaspoon low-sodium soy sauce
1/4	cup tomato paste
1/4	cup water

In small bowl combine spices and vinegar until blended. Then add remaining ingredients and stir until smooth. Makes four 2-tablespoon servings.

Per serving: 20 calories; 0 grams protein; 4 grams carbohydrate; 0 grams fat; 60 milligrams sodium.

Cocktail Sauce

Prepare ketchup as above, then stir in 2 tablespoons prepared horseradish. Makes five 2-tablespoon servings.

Per serving: 20 calories; 0 grams protein; 4 grams carbohydrate; 0 grams fat; 100 milligrams sodium.

DESSERTS

Micro-baked Apple

The old-fashioned comfort of a baked apple in less than 10 minutes! That's no time at all if you bake it while you eat dinner. This is another very adaptable recipe—experiment with spices, other types of apples, pears. The winning combinations are endless.

- 1 red or golden Delicious apple
- 1/3 cup unsweetened apple juice
- 1/2 teaspoon lemon juice
- 1/3 teaspoon vanilla
- 1/4 teaspoon cinnamon

Remove core from apple. Place apple in a small microwaveproof casserole; sprinkle with apple juice, lemon juice, vanilla and cinnamon. Cover with plastic wrap and microwave on High for 3 minutes. Let stand, covered, 5 minutes.
Makes 1 serving.

85 calories; trace protein; 22 grams carbohydrate; trace fat; 1 milligram sodium.

Broiled Banana

A creamy, satisfying dessert as easy as one-two-three! For a Caribbean version, replace the lemon juice with lime, the cinnamon with allspice and top with a splash of rum.

1 ripe banana
1 teaspoon lemon juice
1/4 teaspoon cinnamon

Preheat broiler. Spray a small piece of aluminum foil with non-stick cooking spray. Split the banana in half lengthwise and place on foil on broiler rack. Drizzle with lemon juice and sprinkle on cinnamon. Broil 7 to 9 minutes, until soft and bubbly.

Makes 1 serving.

115 calories; 1 gram protein; 28 grams carbohydrate; 1 gram fat; 1 milligram sodium.

Part III

MAXIMUM METABOLISM: MAKING IT WORK

Chapter 8

THE INNER GAME OF DIETING: THINKING YOURSELF THIN

I T WAS A Monday morning. It was raining. I couldn't get a cab. My receptionist was out sick. And my first patient of the day was going to be a challenge.

Suzanne weighed 135 pounds. She was 5' 5". She wanted to lose about another ten pounds to reach her ideal weight. She also had high blood pressure and had to lose weight to relieve it. By that rainy Monday morning, she had already been on the Maximum Metabolism eating program for three weeks. She had lost thirteen pounds, which I thought was a great success, and her blood pressure was also way down. But she was miserable.

"Doctor, I hate being on this diet. I can't eat all the things I want and all the things I'm used to eating. Worst of all, I'm a gourmet cook. What can I cook when I entertain that will impress people? What can I do? I feel like I'm not really living."

By the time Suzanne had finished complaining, I was almost ready to give up on her. How could I convince her that what she was doing was something that she herself wanted to do, something in her own best interest? Suddenly a light went on in my head and I realized that Suzanne illustrated one of the most important aspects of successful dieting: You need to make a mental as well as a physical change.

"Suzanne," I said, "do you realize that from what you just said to me, there is no way that you can be happy with your life? If you are eating the wrong things, your blood pressure is up, your weight is up and you feel terrible. You told me all about how bad you felt a few weeks ago. And now you've managed to change all that but you feel deprived and unhappy because you're not eating the foods that made you overweight and that originally caused the problem. I thought I solved your problem by giving you an eating program that you could easily stick with, one that would virtually guarantee weight loss. But I only created a new problem. Your problem is not your body—it's your head!" I knew that I had to help Suzanne change the way she thought about dieting.

Needless to say, Suzanne was somewhat taken aback. But I must give her credit: She didn't storm out of my office. She had never thought about her life in quite that way. By her next visit, Suzanne told me she'd thought about what I had said and had made an effort to change her thinking.

I'm telling you Suzanne's story because it makes an absolutely crucial point about how to succeed on the Maximum Metabolism Diet: You need to change the way you think as well as the way you eat.

The premise of Maximum Metabolism is that overweight is not something that happens to you because you have no willpower or because you're lazy or because you have a weak character. At this point in the book it must seem obvious to you that it's the way your body works—your metabolic rate, the effect of certain foods on your hunger and cravings, your need for supplements—that determines your weight. Maximum Metabolism gives you all the ammunition you need to get control of your body and set it on the road to permanent weight loss.

When I first began to work with dieters I focused all my energy on finding a combination of foods and supplements that would guarantee weight loss, eliminate hunger and stop cravings. But as I worked closely with my patients, in workshops, I gradually realized that other factors in their lives were sometimes sabotaging their dieting efforts. A few patients simply needed to know what to eat but most needed help with other aspects of their lives as well. I realized that the best and most effective diet in the world can't help someone who doesn't know what's going on in his or her mind as well as body!

- Barbara could easily stick to a diet when she was safely immersed in her daily routine. But when she traveled, as she had to for her job, she couldn't seem to maintain momentum. In fact, she had trouble with a diet as soon as there was any change in her daily routine.

- Jill would struggle valiantly on her diet but she just couldn't deal with her husband's constant undermining of her efforts. She didn't even *realize* he was undermining her and when she did come to that realization, she was so angry, she couldn't get over it and she certainly couldn't diet.

- Joanne was a great "private dieter." She only got off balance when she had to go to a dinner party or visit a home and then she lost all control.

- Leah was the opposite of Joanne: She was a "public dieter" who would tell everyone she was on a diet and eat nothing when she went out but would regularly binge on ice cream and other sweets the minute she got home.

Over a period of time these patients revealed their emotional problems to me and I became convinced that there

167

was more to dieting than knowing what to eat. You had to learn to *think* about dieting in a new way. I now recognize that you not only need an effective diet; you need to learn *how to diet.* I ultimately adapted some specific techniques that changed my patients' lives: Not only were they able to diet successfully but they also began to meet other challenges in their lives with new confidence.

THE TYRANNY OF LABELS

Before I discuss the psychological concepts that can help you lose weight and see yourself as a thin person, I want you to banish the past. That is, I want you to forget about what you've heard about psychology and weight loss. There are many excellent methods of weight loss that incorporate a psychological approach, but there are also some that are useless and some that are absolutely counterproductive. It's too easy to get all this information confused, and since I want you to begin Maximum Metabolism dieting with positive, clear-eyed optimism and without any of the old-fashioned ideas that may have stymied your past dieting efforts, let's start fresh.

First of all, you should know that there are no overweight personality traits. Researchers love to pin descriptive terms on overweight people in an effort to get at the root cause of obesity. Some of the terms you'll see in journals and even popular books include: depressed, anxious, passive, submissive, defiant, immature, orally fixated, love-starved, self-indulgent, self-punishing, excessively dependent and so on. But the fact is that the latest research demonstrates that these terms are *useless:* None of these traits are any more common among the overweight than among slim people.

Why is this important? Because it's too easy for overweight people to become "victims of labels": If they are told they are depressed or love-starved or self-punishing, they believe that losing weight is out of their control; their problem is a psychological one and they'll probably never lose weight without a great deal of psychological work. Haven't you told yourself at least once or twice that you couldn't diet this month because you're feeling too anxious or stressed? I want you to be liberated from those kinds of thoughts so you can give the Maximum Metabolism program the best chance of success.

Mary was a classic "victim of labels." When she came to see me she wanted help with her food allergies. She was fifty pounds overweight but she never mentioned any desire to lose weight. When I brought up the subject of weight loss in relation to health, Mary told me that of course she would like to lose weight but she didn't think it was possible, at least at this juncture of her life. She had just moved from a midwestern city with her husband and baby and was feeling terribly depressed. She missed her friends and hadn't been able to make new ones. In fact, she had gained thirty pounds in the six months since the move. "Maybe when I'm feeling better, Doctor. I know there's no point in even trying right now. There's no way I could climb out of this depression enough to concentrate on losing weight; I'm too vulnerable."

Now please understand that I had great sympathy for Mary's situation. It's very difficult to take on a self-improvement project when you're feeling depressed. But you can see how Mary's self-diagnosis of depression had effectively stopped her from doing something that could considerably improve her life. She *was* vulnerable: vulnerable to an old-fashioned idea! In fact, Mary did finally lose thirty pounds and is on her way to reaching her goal. As she says: "I was using a label to protect myself. If I was depressed, I was 'off the hook.' No one could expect very much from me. But I'm glad someone made me see what I was doing to myself. I now understand that the wrong food choices were making me fat—not depression. I wish I could convince every over-weight person I see how liberating it is to take this approach."

In telling Mary's story, I don't mean to dismiss the value of psychological understanding and insights. It's just that in most cases overweight did not happen as a result of a psychological deficiency; it happened because your body got off track. You do not need to think of yourself as a "fat person" with a "fat personality"—you are a thin person who is temporarily fat.

THINKING YOURSELF THIN: IT WORKS!

There *is* a technique that has proven very successful for dieters in a variety of situations and it's one that I've used with excellent results. I refer to it as "thinking yourself thin." I think you'll find it a powerful technique that will insure permanent weight loss for you.

This technique first became popular in sports when researchers realized that the way athletes thought could actually improve their skills. This was a revolutionary concept and at first there were many skeptics. But time and again it was demonstrated that if you practiced your *thinking* about, say, your golf stroke you could see as much or more improvement than if you simply got up and swung the club. You had to imagine yourself swinging the club, imagine the perfect arc of the ball, imagine the proper follow-through and then imagine you saw the ball dropping in the cup. The technique itself was fairly simple. And, amazingly, it worked. Statistics proved it. Much to my delight, cognitive restructuring is just as effective for dieters as for athletes.

To "think yourself thin" you must first get away from the idea that you can't control your thoughts. Like Mary, you must accept the fact that *you* are in control.

And while you may not be able to control what goes on in

your life, you are always able to control what goes on in your head!

This seems such a simple concept but it's absolutely crucial to the success of your Maximum Metabolism program. One of my patients told me: "Doctor, I've lost weight and I'm doing well on the diet. In fact, I'm coping with situations that always used to be my downfall. But there's one thing: I just don't ever believe that I will be able to be in a situation where other people are eating and not want to eat myself." My answer to this is simple: If you don't believe you will ever be able to do something, you won't. If you don't believe you'll be able to lose weight, you won't. If you don't believe you will be able to cut down on fat, you won't. The power to do these things begins in your mind. Where else could it begin? No one can make you eat unless they hold a gun to your head and force you to do so and no one can make you lose weight but *you*.

There are two steps to thinking yourself thin: First you need to change the habits of thinking—the habits of thinking "fat"—that you've acquired over the years. Then you must learn new techniques of thinking. You have to learn to substitute "thin" thinking.

You begin this whole process by thinking about what you're thinking about.

If you are awake, your mind is at work. But most people spend no conscious time trying to direct their thoughts. If you learn how to tap into the power of your thoughts, you will discover a source of strength—strength for change and improvement—that you never dreamed was possible!

Your constant inner monologue—thoughts about the weather, where you're going tonight, how your right shoe is tight, whether or not your husband remembered to make reservations for next week—influences your behavior in all areas of your life. Most dieters are unaware that their thoughts are defeating them, particularly when it comes to thoughts about eating.

If you focus on food—what you had for breakfast, what you want to have for lunch, what kind of a snack you'd like to have with a cup of coffee—you'll find that these thoughts influence your eating. Thinking about food will increase your appetite. Thinking about food can make it easier for you to overeat. Remember hyperresponders who experience insulin surges at just the thought of food? You can, in effect, give yourself permission to overeat by thinking about how you'd enjoy a certain meal.

But the opposite is also true: If you direct your thoughts toward eating the right foods, toward getting some exercise, toward accepting yourself as someone who is going to be thin, someone who is proud of his or her body and determination, I promise you that you'll see the difference not only in weight loss but also in an overall improvement in self-esteem.

THE HABIT OF THINKING THIN

Many thought patterns are simply ingrained habits. You don't think about a habit; it's automatic. If you want to channel your thoughts to help you lose weight, you must change your thinking habits. You do this the same way you would change any habit. In fact, behavioral researchers have developed extremely effective methods for changing habits. The techniques I use with my patients are based on these proven methods.

1. *First you must identify the problem.*
You've probably been on a diet before. Chances are you went off it at some point. Why? You wanted to lose weight. You wanted to look better. But something happened and your goals shifted and you suddenly wanted to eat more than you wanted to be thin. How did this happen? If you don't try to understand why, it could happen again.

You must zero in on the negative thought patterns that encourage you to eat. Here is a chart that lists the most common negative thoughts that run through dieters' minds. Please read through and identify those that apply to you. Be honest with yourself about which thoughts you have. Some of my patients identify four or five negative thoughts while others find only one. But at some point in the past, one of these thoughts sabotaged your diet and you need to understand why.

The Very Best Reasons for Being Overweight

1. I'll start dieting again—tomorrow.
2. It's never worked before; why should it now?
3. I'm so overweight it would take forever; so why begin?
4. I don't really care about losing weight.
5. It's always been too hard to lose; there must be something wrong with me.
6. I'm losing too slowly.
7. No one really cares so why bother?
8. Everybody is making this hard for me; I might as well give up.
9. Poor me! I have to give up everything I like.
10. It's so unfair that other people can eat anything they want and I can't.
11. I can't expect my family to change the way they eat because of me.
12. What if I regain some weight? I couldn't stand it after all the work I put into this.
13. What if I don't have enough willpower?
14. I'm so worthless I don't deserve to be thin.
15. It smells/looks so good I can't resist.
16. I'm really starving and I've got to eat.
17. I can't stop thinking about food.
18. If it weren't for my job/kids/husband/schedule I could lose weight.
19. He/she insists that I eat.
20. I deserve a little treat now and again.

21. With my schedule, it's impossible to eat right.
22. I can't let it go to waste.
23. I paid for it; I might as well eat it.
24. I'll never get a chance to eat this again.
25. The holidays come only once a year.
26. My life is too stressful right now to diet.
27. I'm so tired I couldn't possibly cook anything.
28. I've got to eat so I won't get a headache.
29. I can't be expected to stick to my diet under these circumstances.
30. Well, there goes my diet; I might as well give up.

Did some of these thoughts ring a bell with you? Did you ever think about what these thoughts really mean and how they affect your life? Did you ever realize that these habits of thinking could be keeping you from being as thin and as happy as you were meant to be?

Now that you've met the enemy, you can cope with it. You need to take a look at these thoughts. Do they make sense? Are they helping you achieve a goal? Is there any truth in them? The answer, of course, is a resounding no! So let's substitute some thoughts that *are* going to help you and that *are* going to make a positive difference.

2. *Positive self-talk is the core of your new healthy approach to food.*

You need to restructure the inner monologues that subvert your dieting efforts. This is all so simple but it's important! Start to re-think your problem areas. For example, if you are thinking "Poor me, I have to give up almost everything I like", then you have to restructure that thought. What do you really like? Bread and butter? Cookies? Cake? Ice cream? How do you feel when you eat those things? What do those things do to your body and your health and your self-esteem? Do they really make you feel good? Or do they ultimately make you feel out of control and depressed? What is the truth about the things you like? And what about the things you're eating on this diet? Don't they make you feel good? Don't they make you feel like you're in control of your life? Don't you think the result is worth it?

When you come right down to it, it's not really a case of "poor me" at all, is it? So why not stop thinking that way since it's only a sure-fire route to failure. Why not start thinking, "I'm not depriving myself of anything. These foods are really bad for me. I feel much better when I don't eat them."

You see? You have to eliminate your negative talk. You have to harness all that unconscious energy to work for you instead of against you.

Right now focus on each of the negative thoughts that have sabotaged you in the past. Think about why they don't really make sense. Think about how you need to turn that thought around. Think about the most important fact of all: You want to change your eating habits and your want to be healthier and feel better than you ever have before.

Whenever you catch yourself thinking something negative, be prepared to change your inner dialogue to something positive. For example: "I'll never be able to look good in a bathing suit by my vacation next month. I might as well have dessert today." You could replace this negative thought with something like this: "If I have dessert today, I'll only delay when I can look great in a bathing suit. Besides, I already look better than I did two weeks ago. And I feel better than I have in ages. One dessert isn't really worth it."

SUCCESS IS AN ATTITUDE: THE MAXIMUM METABOLISM MIND-BOOSTERS

Now that you've reached a new understanding about the negative thoughts that sabotage your diet, you need a few techniques to ease your passage to success. I think of these techniques as "mental supplements" because, like the vitamin and mineral supplements that give your body a boost, these techniques give you a "mental" boost: They strengthen the attitude you need to be successful at changing your diet.

1. *Recognize that you have a new goal.*

Your Maximum Metabolism goal is to change your eating habits! I can't emphasize this enough. The result of accomplishing your goal will be weight loss. I guarantee you that if you keep your energy focused on changing your eating habits you will lose weight and you will have a much easier time doing so. It's very difficult for some people to make this change in their thinking but it's essential.

Are you the kind of dieter who has begun a number of diets determined to lose ten pounds in a week? Some diets actually encourage this kind of thinking by promising you dramatic, if impossible, results. But how do you feel after the week has passed and you've lost only one pound and are exhausted and irritable? Like a failure.

And what about those daily goals that you become obsessive about? "I'm going to eat nothing all day except for a small salad at lunch." Or: "I'm going to exercise every day for an hour." Maybe you can actually achieve some of these goals but the chances of doing so are dismal at the outset.

The problem with these impossible goals is not the individual failures; it's the extended pattern of failure that becomes difficult to escape.

The scenario goes something like this: You decide to lose thirty pounds by the day of your daughter's wedding in eight weeks. You starve yourself for a week. You're tired and irritable. You can barely cope with all the stresses of wedding planning. You decide it's really not worth it. You'll just find something to wear that looks OK on you. You lose all self-restraint and gain an additional three pounds. You're so disgusted with yourself that you vow to forget all ideas of dieting. A year later, when you begin to think about losing some weight, you remember the last diet you were on and decide to postpone even thinking about it.

You can see how self-defeating impossible goals can be. Rather than deciding to "lose thirty pounds," which is a difficult goal, make your goals positive and short-term. Decide to avoid all unhealthy snacks. Decide to throw out all the fattening treats in your cupboard. Decide to exercise for an extra fifteen minutes today. These are goals that *are* within reach and accomplishing them will give you the kind of positive reinforcement that will spell long-term success.

2. *Change your "fat thinking" by learning to rechannel your negative thoughts.*

When you rechannel your negative thoughts, you'll be working on what's going on *inside* your head—where your bad eating habits start.

Rechanneling your negative thoughts is simply a method of planning ahead for the habits of thinking that keep you from losing weight. I've found that there are three common negative thoughts that cause people to fall off diets:

- "I'm bored."
- "I'm deprived."
- "I'm not losing weight fast enough."

None of these thoughts really makes any sense but that doesn't stop them from having their devastating effect.

The thought that you're bored with your new eating habits, for example, is usually beside the point. One of my patients told me that she got bored after a week or so on every diet she'd ever been on. I asked her what she usually ate when she wasn't dieting. It turned out that she had virtually the same breakfast and the same lunch every day. Her dinners varied but her bedtime snack of ice cream was also repeated at least five times a week. Her unhealthy diet was totally boring!

Be prepared for this negative thought. If you begin to think you're bored, think about what you're eating now and what you used to eat. Remind yourself that being bored is probably an excuse. Think about the positive effects of the good foods you're eating—not only the positive effect of weight loss but also the way you feel in terms of energy, sense of accomplishment, etc.

Thoughts of boredom are often accompanied by thoughts of deprivation. A patient will begin to feel deprived. If this happens to you, follow that thought to its logical conclusion. What do you really mean by "deprived"? Do you feel more "fulfilled" when you go on a cookie binge? When you eat a steak and baked potato slathered with butter? When you have a huge dessert at a fancy restaurant? No! In fact you feel out of control, disappointed in yourself, maybe even a little sick.

If you stop to think about it, these new eating habits are probably making you feel better than ever. Don't you feel more energetic? Doesn't it feel great to feel your clothes loosen? Don't you feel more in control of your life than ever before and haven't you felt this sense of control affecting other aspects of your life, including perhaps work and relationships with others? So don't be tricked into believing you're deprived. Rechannel your negative thoughts into a more positive and accurate attitude. Tell yourself the real truth: that feeling deprived is how you feel when you can't fit into nice clothes and when you can't feel proud of your body.

Being unhappy with the rate of your weight loss is usually a result of focusing solely on weight loss as a goal. It's one of the reasons I recommend that your goal be healthy eating habits instead. If you set your sights on losing a certain number of pounds, I can almost promise you that at some point you will become discouraged. Most patients reach a plateau where their weight loss slows or stops for a period of time. Scientists have yet to arrive at a conclusion as to why this happens but it almost invariably does. I've seen countless patients go for a week with no appreciable weight loss but with a considerable figure change. That is, while they're not losing any pounds, their clothes are getting looser and they look thinner. If you keep your eyes glued to the scale, you may miss the fact that your body *is* changing even if the needle seems stuck.

And what about those people who go for three weeks losing only a pound a week? If your goal is to change your eating habits you will still be having successful weeks. But if your goal is only to "lose weight" you could become discouraged. Though I've never had a patient who lost only a pound a week, I must say that a fifty-two-pound weight loss over a period of a year is something that any dieter could be proud of and, in fact, it's probably more than many people would want to lose!

I hope that it's clear to you now how you must rechannel your negative thoughts by arming yourself with the facts. The facts are positive weapons that will help you stick to your new eating program. Review them regularly.

3. *Learn to Use "Mental Movies."*
Remember those negative thoughts that have always stymied you in the past? Get used to practicing an exercise I call "mental movies" to banish these thoughts once and for all. Mental movies are amazingly effective because when you see yourself doing what you want to do, you're on your way to doing it.

Lisa, a freelance writer, told me that she found it almost impossible to stick to her diet when she visited her mother. She said that she recognized from my list of "The Very Best Reasons for Being Overweight" that her mother encouraged her to eat and she couldn't resist; it just didn't seem worth it to oppose her. I asked Lisa what she thought about before she got to her mother's house. She said: "All I can think about is how awful it will be and how I'll revert to a child the minute I walk in the door. I'll give in and eat something I don't want and I'll feel awful and angry. And when I get home I'll feel even angrier and I probably won't speak to my mother for two weeks even though she won't understand why."

Lisa obviously gave a lot of thought to her visit but all of it was negative. I taught her how to substitute a positive mental movie.

Now Lisa has an altogether different approach to visits with her mother. When she thinks about them in advance, she doesn't focus on food. Instead, she runs a "mental movie" in her mind about how nice it will be to see her mother and what things they'll have to talk about. She calls her mother in advance and suggests they go to a restaurant that Lisa knows will serve things appropriate to her diet. She reminds her mother that she wants to stick to her new eating plan so she shouldn't prepare any treats for her. Lisa sees herself refusing with good cheer if her mother does prepare a treat or she sees herself taking the treat home to give to a neighbor and explaining how much her friend will enjoy the gift. Lisa can now visit her mother without bad feelings and without going off her diet.

One of the most common pitfalls of dieting among my patients is restaurant dining. Mental movies are wonderfully effective in transforming your restaurant experience. I used mental movies myself when I gave up drinking. I ate out a lot and realized that abstaining from drinking in a restaurant was my biggest challenge.

Your dining-out mental movie should go something like this. First you imagine yourself entering the restaurant. You see yourself checking your coat and being seated at your table. You ask the waiter to remove the bread. You see yourself ordering a nonalcoholic drink. You imagine the conversation. You look forward to the broiled fish or chicken you know that particular restaurant prepares so well. You see yourself telling the waiter not to bring you a dessert menu and asking for fruit to end the meal. The most important part of the movie is the "emotional sound track": You're having fun, you're enjoying yourself! And you're sticking to your new healthy eating patterns.

Mental movies are enormously helpful when you know that you are going to face a diet challenge. A child's birthday party, a holiday, a dinner out can challenge your diet and you need to "think yourself thin" before the event. Run a movie in your mind's eye of you at the event eating appropriate foods and enjoying them. Visualize yourself refusing a tempting dessert or a piece of bread with good humor and a feeling of confidence. When the time comes, you'll find these actions much easier to carry out: You've already practiced them in your mind. You really will be amazed at how these mental movies can give you confidence and encouragement.

4. *Be your own best friend.*

This is a simple technique that has been a revelation for many of my patients. Here's how it works. When you have a dieting problem or challenge or even a dieting setback, talk to yourself about it in a constructive way. Imagine that your best friend is presenting the problem to you. Think about the advice you would give to your friend and then take the advice to heart.

It's amazing how hard we are on ourselves and how readily we can become confused and discouraged. But the path out of the woods is often right there in our own heads.

Barbara, a surgical nurse, told me what a difference this technique had made to her. "I used to fuss and worry endlessly about my husband's cooking. It's not what you think: He's a great cook—too great a cook; I was twenty-five pounds overweight. Because my hours are so crazy, he winds up cooking at least half of our meals. And when he didn't cook, he'd insist on giant hunks of meat and potatoes running with butter. My husband is one of those types who can never gain weight no matter what he eats. I would start fights about him spending so much time cooking. I would come home late for dinner. I would come home early for dinner and then be angry at him when I overate. But I never really discussed the problem with him. I guess I didn't even have it straight in my own mind.

"Then I followed your advice. I pretended a friend had come to me with the same problem. I would tell her that if she really wanted to lose weight, she'd have to discuss it with her husband. She'd have to tell him that he's a terrific cook but it was too hard for her to resist those great meals. They'd have to make a new arrangement about meals—one that would allow her to lose weight.

"Well, my husband was very cooperative about it. He said that he never really believed I was serious about losing weight but he thought it was wonderful that I was making the effort and he'd do all he could to support me. He still has to have his meat a few times a week but I passed along some Maximum Metabolism recipes and now he's making fabulous *diet* meals for me. He never snacks in front of me and he keeps telling me how great I look. And I guess I do. I only have six more pounds to go."

You know that you are going to face challenges on your diet; every dieter does. Try to anticipate what a few of them might be right now and think about what you would tell your best friend if he or she told you about that particular problem. It's amazing how clearly we can sometimes see the problems of others while we feel totally confused and trapped by our own.

Whenever you feel yourself going in circles about any aspect of your diet, try to be your own best friend. I think you'll be delighted with the results.

How to Survive the Worst Diet Days

There will always be days that are a dieter's nightmare. You're late for work and couldn't eat anything at home. Should you just grab a doughnut and coffee? Or you have to entertain at lunch and the client suggests a restaurant, a terrific Italian place that specializes in old-fashioned Southern Italian cooking. Should you break down just this once and have that lasagna that you haven't had in nearly six weeks? Or maybe you had a fight with your boss in the afternoon. You'll show him; you'll have a big piece of cake at your coffee break. And now your husband calls to say he's invited two colleagues to dinner. That does it: there's nothing in the house you can serve that's appropriate to your eating plan and would also pass as "company" food. And you have no time to shop after work. Can this diet be saved?

Yes! Here are some techniques that my patients have used with resounding success, on their worst-nightmare diet days as well as when they face minor diet challenges:

• *Keep your sense of humor.* This is your life! This is not a rehearsal to be gotten through with gritted teeth so you can get on to the "real" thing. You will invariably encounter difficult, if not impossible, situations. The common reaction is to grimace, do a slow burn and/or look for someone to blame. You are not a "bad" person if you do this—we are, after all, human—but if you think about it, you really are wasting a lot of energy.

I was interested to read recently about a study on executives under great stress. While all worked through the period of stress, about half became sick immediately after the stress had passed. Those who didn't all shared certain traits: They were able to keep a sense of humor about their work, regarded life as a challenge and saw problems as *inevitable*.

A patient of mine, June, told me that she had experienced a dieter's nightmare day similar to the one I described above. By the time work was over and she had to face the evening she was furious. Furious at herself because she had overeaten at lunch; furious at her boss because of their disagreement; furious at her husband because he had, to her way of thinking, ruined both her day and her diet. Then, on the way home, she began to think about her day. In a way, it really was kind of amusing. She began to see it as an *I Love Lucy* segment on dieting. What would Lucy serve for dinner? What would little Ricky have up his sleeve to further sabotage her day? After thinking this way for a while, she said that her whole attitude changed. She even felt a bit silly for reacting so strongly to her setbacks. She felt especially bad, she told me, for being so angry at her husband.

By the time June got home, she was in a totally different frame of mind and she had figured out a carry-out dinner she could order that would suit her eating goals and also please her guests. Best of all, she said, her good humor made the evening fun for herself and everyone else. And, despite her lapse earlier in the day, she did manage to stick to her eating plan.

Since she described her experience to a group of Maximum Metabolism dieters, others have told me that they found the *I Love Lucy* method of keeping their sense of humor particularly effective.

- *Learn to be flexible.* You can subvert your best efforts at dieting by being a perfectionist. Many overweight people seize upon the smallest lapse and magnify it to the proportions of a major failure. This is terribly self-defeating. One of the goals of thinking yourself thin is to learn to be more flexible about your mistakes. You need to learn to recognize a lapse as a simple isolated event, not a signal to give up. A lapse does not indicate failure; it's your *reaction* to a lapse that counts.

Try to be as understanding with yourself as you would be with a best friend. If you go to a party and can't resist the bowl of peanuts at your elbow, use it as a learning experience. Don't for one minute think about how "bad" you were. Instead see what you can learn from your mistake. How could you avoid such a lapse in the future? Should you have a snack before the party? Should you make a point of never sitting near food? Should you make a point of sipping some seltzer to keep your hands busy?

The point is that you need to find your own unique, effective solutions to the ongoing challenges your diet will present.

• *Think of your diet as an opportunity and a challenge, not a punishment.* Maggie, a children's librarian, told me she thought she'd never been able to diet successfully because she considered diets something that "bad" people had to endure. If she was "good" she wouldn't have to be on a diet. In fact, it took a few weeks before Maggie could begin a consultation with me without saying "I was very good this week, Doctor."

A diet is not a punishment. Don't look upon it as a prison that excludes food. You are not going to eat "good" foods; you're going to eat the "right" foods. You are going to begin to feel like a different person. You are going to begin to think like a thin person. You are going to begin to look like a different person. People around you are going to notice a change in you. By changing your old eating habits you really have the opportunity to change your life!

• *Learn success from your mistakes.* This is another simple concept that completes the cycle of improvement and locks in good results. I hope that most of the time you will have a positive reaction to negative self-talk and eating triggers.

You should then reflect on your success and take pleasure in it.

If you get through a family holiday without eating improperly, you deserve congratulations. If you go on vacation and manage to eat healthful foods and get some exercise, you have achieved a real success. On the other hand, there will be times when you fail. You'll overeat at a dinner party. You'll lose control and buy a cookie from a vendor at a fair. The crucial part of a failure is your reaction to it! If you tell yourself you've failed and there's no reason to keep trying to diet, you've lost. A patient told me that her two-year-old son, when informed that the dog had stolen a loaf of bread off the counter and eaten it, said: "I can't believe it; let's shoot her!" We can laugh at this reaction from a child who doesn't understand what he's saying but if we think about it for a minute, we can recognize that kind of overreaction in our own response to failure.

If you put failure in perspective; if you tell yourself that you made a mistake and try to understand why it happened and how you can avoid such situations in the future, you've achieved real success. If you shoot the dog, you've accomplished nothing.

It's like the follow-through in sports: you have to complete the cycle of activity so you understand what's happening. That way you repeat the good and avoid the bad. It's an integral step in the behavioral changes that will help you maintain your weight loss for years to come.

Chapter 9

DIETING IN THE REAL WORLD: OVERCOMING SOCIAL SABOTAGE

YOU'VE WANTED TO lose weight for a long time. There have been so many times when you couldn't even get started. And there have been a few times when you did enjoy some success. You lost five or ten or fifteen pounds. But then, one day, you went off your diet. For some reason, a moment came along when it seemed more desirable to eat than to stick to your diet. Why? You didn't really think about it at the time. You just went off the diet and in a few weeks, you'd gained back all the weight you'd lost. How did it happen? What made you want to eat again? What made you willing to sacrifice what you'd already accomplished?

In many cases, dieters fail because of their diets: They experience terrible cravings or hunger. But you know that on the Maximum Metabolism Diet that won't happen to you. We've also learned how to handle the negative thoughts that can weaken a dieter's resolve. You're home free . . . right? Well, almost. There is still another powerful factor that can encourage you to abandon your diet no matter how successful you are, no matter how much weight you've lost, no matter how good you feel and how much you want to continue.

What force could possibly be so destructive and so powerful? It comes disguised as the other people in your life: your children, boss, lover, the stranger who sits next to you on the dinner flight. It may be a spouse who urges you to try dessert at a fancy restaurant, a friend who wants you to share a "forbidden" treat, a mother who pressures you to eat because "you look too thin."

Whoever is involved in encouraging you to abandon your diet—even if in the form of the unspoken pressure of strangers at a cocktail party—represents a force that you can't tolerate. And the most important thing to know about social pressures is this: Other people are not the problem; they are simply the excuse. *You* are the problem because you haven't learned to cope with social pressures.

As I said before, no one can make you eat without holding a gun to your head. And when you tell yourself that it's not your fault you ate the piece of cake at the dinner party (the hostess would have been so disappointed) or that you ate those sweet rolls at the family breakfast (everyone else was munching away and you didn't want them to think you have to worry so much about your weight), you're simply making excuses.

I don't mean to be hard on you when I say this. It's extremely difficult to withstand social pressure. I know from my own experience with struggling to change my habits. It's tough, but you have to learn to do it if you want to succeed in losing weight once and for all. Those other people are always going to be in your life and you need to develop the skills to deal effectively with them, as well as with what goes on in your mind when you're under social pressure. How do people "make" you eat? How can you stop this from happening so you can be free to become a successful social dieter? Social situations are the cause of many of my patients' past diet failures and they have found that learning how to be a social dieter has paid off handsomely in their continued weight loss.

There's another aspect to social dieting that's very positive: Other people can be an enormous help to you if you know how to recruit them into your camp. In fact, other people in your life are such a powerful force for good or bad that they can make or break your dieting efforts. By learning to harness their support as well as avoiding their negative pressures, you'll have a powerful weapon in your battle against overweight.

Coping with People Pressure

How vulnerable are you to pressure from other people? Some of us can step aside from the crowd and cry "The Emperor has no clothes!" but most of us are affected by what people around us are thinking and doing. Here's a list of situations that will help you recognize some of the social factors that may make dieting difficult for you.

- "I can't expect other people to want to help me lose weight."

- "If I'm at a restaurant I can't order diet food or my fellow diners will feel uncomfortable."

- "If someone else is paying for my meal, I really shouldn't insult them by eating light."

- "If I have company, I really have to feed them well" [which most people understand to mean high-calorie foods].

- "If I'm invited to dinner, it's rude not to eat most of the meal."

- "Speaking to the hostess before the dinner about what's going to be served is rude."

- "Sometimes if someone pressures me to do something, I resist even if it's a good idea."

- "If changing my weight makes someone I love uncomfortable, I don't think I can do it."

- "If others are eating, I feel I have to join them."

- "If I'm at a party or holiday celebration, I'm simply not strong enough to resist eating."

- "If someone is trying to be nice to me, it's not really right to say no."

- "If someone has prepared food especially for me, it's not polite to refuse it."

- "Sometimes it's very difficult for me to speak up for what I need or want."

- "I often put my needs second rather than hurt another person's feelings."

Did you find yourself answering yes to quite a few of these questions? If so, you are vulnerable to social pressure. This isn't really negative, however. Remember that people can help as well as hinder your dieting efforts. But you do need to learn how to resist the bad pressures and encourage the good ones.

People who are very vulnerable to social pressure—and most of my overweight patients seem to be—have two particular problems: They don't believe that what they want is important. And they don't know how to say no.

If you work on these two areas you'll find that not only is it easier to lose weight, you'll also be more confident and successful in other areas of your life.

Monica told me that she recognized herself in many of the "people pressures" situations I described above. She found it nearly impossible to refuse food in any social situation. "I never really thought about it before but I guess what it comes down to is that I want people to like me and so I feel that if they offer me food, they won't like me if I refuse. It took a lot of work before I really believed that they would like me even if I didn't eat with them. Now I'm able to say no and feel comfortable. I know that liking myself is, in the long run, more important than worrying about other people liking me."

If other people don't like you because you refuse food, it's because they want to justify their own overeating. I've found this to be true almost all the time. People who put real pressure on you to eat want to overeat themselves and they somehow feel better if you overeat too. But most people really don't care if you eat or not! If they have any reaction at all to your refusing food, it's one of respect, admiration or even envy because they can't do it themselves.

Yet knowing that other people don't really care what you eat (unless they have their own eating problem) is only a side issue: What really matters is that you need to acknowledge that your goal—sticking to the diet—is important to you. I suggest that patients repeat this thought to themselves as a background to their mental movie if they are about to face a diet challenge involving others: "Sticking to my diet is important to me and I'm going to do it!"

Timothy told me an interesting story about his last sales meeting. He had already lost fifteen pounds but he had another twenty-five to lose. These meetings were usually high-spirited events with overeating and drinking the norm. But Tim decided in advance that this year would be different for him. He spoke with the hotel as soon as he got there to ask about light food and they were happy to oblige. But when the other salespeople saw Tim abstaining from the steak and ice cream cake as well as the alcohol, they began to tease him. As he said, "If it had been a year ago, I don't think I would have been able to handle it. But I kept telling everyone that I was doing so well on this diet and I was going to stick with it because it was really important to me. I didn't waver and I was really proud of myself. The funny thing was that five people came up to me during the course of the meetings and asked me about the diet and what I was eating and how I managed to have so much willpower. I really felt like they saw me in a new light. I also got a lot of compliments about how I looked. It was a real turnaround for me as far as my diet is concerned and personally too."

And what about saying no? It's hard for most of us in many situations and it's terribly difficult for overweight people who feel they are under pressure, real or imagined, from others. Like most skills, it simply involves practice.

Most of us think that we should know how to handle such situations automatically. But in fact, social skills are learned and the more we practice them, the more adept we become. I tell all my patients to practice saying no in mental movies, particularly when they anticipate a diet challenge.

The most difficult social situation seems to be a dinner party at which the hostess urges you to eat. You have to be flexible in this situation. If the hostess is an old friend, you can call her in advance and tell her you're dieting. I don't think it's appropriate, unless you're dealing with a very good friend or family member, to expect to have a special meal prepared for you.

If you don't know your hostess, you can play it by ear. You first must feel comfortable refusing with good grace. A simple "That looks wonderful but I'll pass" or "I just couldn't but thanks . . . you're a terrific cook" will usually work. Sometimes it helps to turn attention elsewhere: "I'm really full but perhaps Bob would like some more . . ."

Occasionally you'll find yourself in a situation where the hostess virtually insists you eat. My patients have told me that the most effective refusal includes a health "excuse." As Walter told me: "I thought this woman would climb over the table and start spooning chocolate soufflé down my throat. After three refusals I finally said 'The truth is it looks fabulous and I'd love to have some but I've been having some health problems and my doctor says that I can't eat chocolate.' It worked. Now I use that excuse whenever someone is really pressuring me. If they inquire about my health problem, I tell them it's high cholesterol. Not many people feel comfortable arguing with a medical excuse."

Another patient told me that her husband persisted in serving her ice cream in the evening while they watched TV even though he was well aware that she was dieting. He simply didn't want to eat alone. Finally one night she thanked him for the ice cream and went to the sink and emptied the contents down the disposal. It was the last time he encouraged her to eat ice cream.

You may have to be creative when you say no, especially if it involves other peoples' habits. For example, Linette tells how she used to have a pizza every Wednesday with friends. She couldn't insist everyone in the group diet but there was nothing available at the pizza place that was appropriate to her own new eating plan. Finally she called her friends and told them that she thought it might be fun to try another restaurant for a change and mentioned one where she knew she could find simple broiled fish and chicken. Much to her delight, her friends were happy with the change and glad she'd suggested it; they had been getting bored with the pizza routine.

When you change unhealthy eating patterns, especially where others are involved, you must remember that what you want is to lose weight and that what *you* want matters. You might even find, as Marjorie did, that friends become converts. Her office friends, who used to lunch together regularly, are now dieting along with her and have become allies and supporters. It seems that they'd all wanted to lose weight but just didn't have the impetus to get started. Marjorie has lost twenty-two pounds and her three friends have all lost too—one lost eighteen pounds. Marjorie gave them the boost they needed and it's changed their lives.

STRATEGIES FOR SOCIAL DIETING

If you're going to succeed in sticking to your new eating program in a social situation you have to plan ahead. You have to do mental movies and practice saying no so that you can turn a diet challenge into a diet triumph.

If you're going to a party, have a snack and drink something like seltzer in advance to make it easier to resist fattening treats. Don't stand near the peanut bowl. Keep your hands full with a drink of seltzer or water. If necessary, disappear to the bathroom when the birthday cake is served. The point is to know in advance what you're going to do. Don't try to make the decision after you've had a drink and no dinner and your hostess is passing you the barbecued chicken wings.

One patient told me that she's gotten in the habit of bringing along her own vegetables when she visits friends for lunch or dinner. Her friends have been so understanding that now she doesn't give it a second thought. She just ducks into the kitchen to steam them and then uses them as the basis for her meal. If the hostess is serving something appropriate like turkey, she'll add that to her vegetables. But even if there's nothing else for her to eat, she still feels satisfied with her large plate full of colorful veggies.

Another patient reported that he and his wife have changed their favorite restaurant. They used to go to a charming neighborhood Italian restaurant where the food was great but high in fat. They now go to a Japanese restaurant where he can easily eat a delicious meal that is low in fat and additives and where his wife enjoys the food too. Of course, some patients have told me that they've found ways of picking through the menus of favorite restaurants so that they can eat healthfully and well. Remember: You can always ask the restaurant to prepare chicken or fish for you simply—broiled, with no sauce. Most restaurants today are happy to oblige.

How to Recruit Allies in the Diet Wars

If you want to lose weight and keep it off, you're going to need the help of others. It is possible to lose weight entirely on your own but it's much more difficult. Enlisting social support gives you strength when you need it as well as a kind of insurance that others care about your efforts. It will also do a great deal to guarantee your long-term success. There are a few techniques that will help you rally those around you to your cause.

• First: Be specific! Some of my patients have said that they've tried to get spouses, friends or children to help them lose weight in the past but without success. When I pressed them for details—what did they ask from their supporters?—their answers were usually vague. It sounds obvious at first: You simply want someone to support you in your efforts to lose weight. But what does that really mean? People won't know how to help you unless you tell them.

You must tell your family and friends what you're trying to do. Explain to them the premise of the Maximum Metabolism Diet. It might be useful to have them read the beginning of this book so they can understand the theory of it. They need to know, especially if they have witnessed past dieting attempts that have ended in failure, that this time things will be different.

Explain to them that you need some very specific help: You need your supporters to respect your efforts to avoid fattening foods by not offering them to you and/or not eating them in your presence. If they must eat potato chips while watching TV, ask them to do it when you're not around. If they must keep fattening snacks in the house, perhaps they can make them ones you don't like. They shouldn't tempt you with high-fat treats as a "reward" for your efforts. You can't expect to change the way your family eats overnight, since this will breed only resentment. But you can ask for their good-natured cooperation in avoiding high-fat foods. Ultimately they'll benefit too.

- Tell your supporters that they are not expected to become "food police." Lisa told me that every time she tried to diet her mother watched every bite she took and commented on its calorie content. Naturally this drove Lisa crazy and became a source of great friction in the household. Moreover, Lisa wound up eating more out of constant irritation. Spouses are often guilty of this pattern. One, perhaps already guilty for being overweight, will either ridicule the efforts of the other to lose or become so obsessed with "helping" that they stymie genuine efforts to change.

  Your supporters should understand that negative comments relating to food are counterproductive. Their motto should be "If you can't be positive, be quiet."

- Ask your supporters to help you focus on fun, not food. Remember when we talked about thinking yourself thin and how what goes on in your mind can dramatically affect your weight loss? This creates a marvelous opportunity for your supporters to offer real help. Ask them to help you focus your thoughts and energy on things other than food. This can be a real challenge because so much of what we consider fun includes food: celebratory dinners, friendly lunches, a companionable ice cream cone after shopping. You'll need some help with thinking of activities that get you out of the kitchen and into something engrossing. Perhaps just a walk in the evening when you used to snack in front of the TV. Or a movie instead of a dinner out. Or dance lessons or a course you can take together.

Richard told me that he did all his snacking in the evening—he just couldn't seem to get through till bedtime without wandering into the kitchen numerous times. In his first week on the Maximum Metabolism Diet, he and his wife subscribed to a film festival at their local college. They loved the activity: It became a sort of "date night" for them. They became so interested in it that they rented other films by directors they particularly enjoyed to watch at home.

As Richard says: "I no longer spend the evening thinking about how much ice cream is left in the container. And as I've lost weight, my wife and I have become closer. It's almost like we were dating again. I guess because we have this shared activity that we both enjoy so much. And of course I look and feel better than I have in years and I can't tell you how much that's helped our relationship. I've already lost eight pounds but I must tell you that right now, with my life so improved, the weight loss seems like a bonus of the diet, not the goal."

• Share your success with your supporters. Tell them what your goals are. Most people think their goal should be seen as number of pounds lost, but I think it's far more effective to share a goal that is smaller and more specific. For example, tell people that your goal this week is no evening snacks that aren't on the Maximum Metabolism Diet. Or your goal is to walk for fifteen blocks during your lunch hour three times a week. Make your goals positive rather than negative. When you've achieved a goal, share the good news. Let your supporters share your pleasure and enthusiasm and take their encouragement seriously.

Some patients have asked, "How can I tell someone to praise me and then believe it when they do?" The fact is that the people in your life have a powerful influence on you. If they truly want you to lose weight they will be genuine in their praise: They simply need to be reminded that the praise and encouragement are valuable to you. And they are!

Chapter 10

Maximizing Your Success: the best real-life dieting tips

THERE SEEMS TO BE a little voice in all of us that appears when we're trying to change. It says "Test yourself! Prove you're strong!" It's the voice that encourages you to go to the doughnut shop with a friend. It's the one that tells you it's OK to buy those cookies; they're for the kids. It's the one that encourages you to eat with friends "just to be sociable"— even though you're not hungry. It's the one that prompts you to order dessert in that great French restaurant: "How often do you go out anyhow? You'd be foolish not to try just one bite to see how it tastes."

Sometimes we just can't resist being hard on ourselves. But dieting is no time to test your character. It's a simple point, but I want you to let it sink in: *Make dieting easy for yourself!* Don't put yourself in difficult situations. Make your environment work for you.

MAKE YOUR WORLD "LITE"

One of the reasons that spas are so successful at helping people lose weight is that they put them in a totally support-ive environment. No cookies in the cupboard. No coffee breaks with honey-dipped doughnuts. No cooking for the family. No office parties. If we could all check into a spa for a month, I'm sure we'd all lose weight. It's easy when you don't have to make any decisions. But that's also why clinics and spas have such a dismal long-term success record. As soon as you go home you're faced with all those temptations you used to succumb to and you immediately revert to old eating patterns.

I want you to take the best features of a spa and incorpo-rate them into your *daily* life. If you do, I promise that you'll achieve both short- and long-term diet success.

Make your kitchen a dieter's heaven rather than a dieter's hell. Eliminate all the food items that you shouldn't eat. I'm sure you know what this means. If you have a box of saltines that you think are totally innocent, fine. But if you're the kind of person (and you know if you are) who at one sitting can eat half a box of saltines spread with peanut butter or jam, get rid of them! The same goes for the peanut butter and/or jam. If, like many people, you must keep certain foods around for other people—say your kids will eat noth-ing but peanut-butter sandwiches—then try to keep those items in a special place, perhaps a separate cabinet. Tell yourself and the rest of your family that that cabinet is out of bounds for you. Once you get the junk out, you'll be safe from those midnight terrors that afflict us all. I don't have a weight problem, but I'm very serious about eating nutritious food. I don't keep any kind of junk in my kitchen. Yet every now and again I rampage through the cabinets, muttering to myself, looking for a goodie. At those times, I'd eat anything I could get my hands on—peanuts, ice cream, potato chips, chocolate-chip cookies. Nothing would be safe. And I think of myself as a disciplined person! When I finally sit down with a piece of fruit, it's only because there's no alternative. I want you to create a kitchen where there are no alternatives.

Keep handy those snack foods—primarily fruits—that are on the Maximum Metabolism Diet, so that if you have the urge to nibble you'll have something right at hand that's good for you. One of my patients told me how she always keeps fresh fruit at hand. She even travels with two fruit snacks in her handbag. Keep stocked up on seltzer or club soda: A glass of plain seltzer or club soda with a squeeze a lemon or lime can be surprisingly satisfying when you want something to drink or even as a substitute for a snack.

Your next stop is the supermarket. Never shop when you're hungry or tired. Try not to shop with small children. Make a shopping list at home and stick to it; don't buy on impulse or cram the refrigerator with unnecessary temptations. Learn to read labels. That cereal you may be buying because you think it's high in fiber may have a great deal of sugar in it. Learn about the fat content of foods. Some items that you may think are innocent could be loaded with fat. Here's a breakdown of a cereal label from the University of California's Berkeley Wellness Letter that I'm sure you'll find useful.

A FOOD LABEL LEXICON*

The language of food labeling, like that of diplomacy, sometimes obscures as much as it reveals. It is bad enough that some foods display no nutrition or ingredient information at all, but some of the information that *is* provided on labels can lead astray even the most savvy consumer. Just consider, a food labeled "sugar-free" or "light" can be chock-full of calories, one "with no salt added" can be loaded with sodium, and a "natural" food can contain many artificial ingredients.

A recent FDA survey found that 68% of Americans who read food labels do so primarily to avoid or limit certain ingredients—most often sodium, saturated fat, cholesterol, sugar, and additives. Nutrition labeling is out of sync with these concerns, responding instead to earlier concerns about vitamin, mineral, and protein deficiencies. Just last year sodium was made a mandatory part of nutrition labels. The other sought-after information seldom appears among the nutrition statistics. You have to know how to read between the lines.

* Reprinted by permission of: *University of California, Berkeley Wellness Letter*, P.O. Box 10922, Des Moines, IA 50340. © Health Letter Associates, 1987

No legal meaning. Product can still contain preservatives, artificial flavoring, and other additives. When comparing brands, make sure serving sizes are the same.

This number must be within 20% of the actual calorie count. Thus a serving of this granola can contain anywhere from 104 to 156 calories.

Amount of saturated and unsaturated fatty acids as well as cholesterol must be listed if health claims are made about them on the package.

These eight nutrients must be listed. Listing of other nutrients is optional, unless they have been added or a claim is made for them. Listed amounts don't account for any losses that may occur during cooking or preparation.

Ingredients are listed in descending order according to weight. This gives you no idea how much of any ingredients is actually used. Standardized foods don't have to list ingredients.

Specific flavors, colors (except Yellow no. 5), and spices don't have to be listed by name; general terms like this are allowed. If you are allergic to some of these, write to food manufacturers to find out which ones they use.

BHT stands for butylated hydroxytoluene, a common preservative in cereals and other foods. Preservatives, thickening agents, emulsifiers, and other additives must be listed on labels. Most of those used today are safe, but a few, such as sulfites, pose health risks for some people. Others, including BHT, are under continuing review.

GRANOLA CEREAL
ALL NATURAL

NUTRITION INFORMATION

SERVING SIZE 1 OUNCE
SERVINGS PER PACKAGE 16

Calories	130
Protein	3g
Carbohydrates	16g
Fat	6g
Sodium	95mg

PERCENTAGE OF U.S. RDA

Protein	4
Vitamin A	*
Vitamin C	*
Thiamine	6
Riboflavin	2
Niacin	2
Calcium	2
Iron	4

*Contains less than 2% U.S. RDA of this nutrient.

INGREDIENTS: Rolled oats, brown sugar, corn syrup, sugar, raisins, peanuts, honey, nonfat dry milk, salt, vegetable oil (one or more of the following: soybean, hydrogenated palm, and/or coconut oil), artificial and natural flavors, preservative BHT, MSG.

Sugars, fiber, and complex carbohydrates are lumped together under carbohydrates. A separate fiber listing is optional; it must be listed if a claim is made about it. There are no regulations concerning fiber labeling. Consumer groups have asked the FDA to make dietary fiber a mandatory part of standard labeling.

To figure out what percentage of calories comes from fat, multiply the grams of fat by 9 (calories in a gram of fat) and divide by the total number of calories. A serving of this granola gets 42% of its calories from fat: 6 times 9 equals 54 fat calories, divided by 130 total calories equals .42, or 42%. That's a lot, since most cereals are low in fat.

The U.S. RDA for calcium is 1,000 mg per day, so 2% is only 20 mg.

"Sugar" means sucrose (table sugar) on a label. But sugar comes in many forms, and they are listed separately, like the brown sugar, corn syrup, and honey seen here. When these are added up, sugar may actually be the predominant ingredient.

Soybean is the only unsaturated oil here. Since palm and coconut oils, which are highly saturated, usually cost less, they are used in many foods.

Monosodium glutamate, a flavor enhancer and a source of sodium. Sodium is found in at least 70 compounds used in foods besides salt, including baking soda (sodium bicarbonate).

Plan Ahead!

You *must* plan ahead if you're going to succeed on the Maximum Metabolism diet. Your biggest downfalls will occur when you've failed to plan and find yourself in a situation where you wing it. For example, you've gotten home from work late and there's nothing to eat. Well, there is lettuce and other salad fixings and there's a frozen chicken breast, but you're starving and you must have something *now*. So you wolf down half a loaf of bread that you toast and slather with butter and cinnamon, since it's the only thing you can make instantly. Sound familiar? You can't afford to eat this way any longer.

I've made it easier than ever for you to plan ahead by including sample restaurant meals and "carry-out" or deli meals in the Maximum Metabolism diet. You'll find these meals will make it much easier for you to stick to the diet. Here are some other specific tips that will help:

Plan your meals a day or two in advance. It becomes routine within a week or so. You should also have the makings for one emergency meal on hand for those times when your schedule changes unexpectedly. This kind of planning ahead will also make your shopping trips more efficient. If you work outside the home, make it a rule never to leave the house in the morning without knowing what you're going to have that evening for dinner. If you're at home all day, make sure you know before lunch what your dinner will be. As Maryanne, a stock analyst, told me: "I used to think that I should be able to just toss something together when I got home from work—something simple and stir-fried that would be low in calories and quick and delicious. Well, in fact in theory I could do this, but I never planned what exactly it would be. So I would get home late and nothing would seem really appetizing, and of course I was tired, and so I'd finally just get carry-out delivered from the deli or the Chinese restaurant in the neighborhood. After a year of this, I'd put on eighteen pounds. Now that I plan my dinners I eat much better, I've already lost twelve pounds and I don't feel defeated, which is the way I always felt for not eating better, particularly at night."

One of my patients told me that she prepares extra-large portions of vegetables at night. The next day she uses the leftover vegetables in a salad by adding lettuce and other greens. Another patient cooks a large pot of soup on Sunday—black bean is his favorite—to eat during the week.

Whenever possible, cook early in the day when you're not likely to be tired or hungry. Many patients have told me that if they have to cook for others or even when they cook for themselves, it's much easier to do so in the morning. If they cook at dinnertime, they do too much snacking and sampling. If a meal is virtually finished and just needs to be heated or assembled for dinner, the temptation to snack is eliminated.

Most people find it easier to resist temptation just after breakfast. Suzanne, a magazine editor, told me: "This rule of cooking in the morning made all the difference to me. I don't do the actual cooking in the morning because I have to leave for work. But I do get up about fifteen minutes early so I can do most of the preparation. Because the meals on the diet are simple to prepare, I find I can get most everything ready while I listen to the morning news shows. Then once I get home, my dinner is ready in no time. I can't tell you what a difference this has made to me. I used to consume about 500 calories before I ever sat down to eat anything. And I usually wasn't very hungry by the time my dinner was ready!"

Change a tempting environment. For example, in a restaurant, ask the waitress not to bring any bread or to take it away if it's already there. If you're flying, call the airline ahead to order a special meal; the fruit plates are usually good. If you're served a dessert at a banquet, put salt on it before you lose your resolve. If you visit friends who are eager to put out some cookies or cake, tell them that you're dieting and would really appreciate either a piece of fruit or perhaps some plain seltzer or club soda. It's even better to let someone know in advance that you won't want any snacks. Or bring along your own seltzer and piece of fruit.

One of my patients—a chocolate salesman, believe it or not—told me about how certain supermarkets bake fresh cookies in the deli department because they know people will smell the aroma and make a beeline for the deli counter for a cookie or two. Be prepared for these situations. Find a supermarket that doesn't bake on the premises if this will be your downfall.

Chapter 11

BACKSLIDING AND INTERRUPTIONS: HOW TO GET BACK ON TRACK

JOAN HAD LOST thirty pounds and still had another five to lose. One day while shopping at a mall she passed a cookie shop. She bought a warm chocolate-chip cookie and ate it. This triggered an eating binge that lasted nearly a week, after which she'd gained back eleven pounds.

After six months, Lucille had reached her target weight. She was delighted with her new figure and renewed energy. But she gradually began to relax her demands upon herself. She was tired of dieting and so she would have "just one" dessert and would skip exercise "just this once" until she was rarely exercising and snacking frequently. Within three months she had regained all the weight she'd lost plus an additional four pounds.

Jack had lost ten pounds: half of his desired weight loss. He was feeling terrific for the first time in five years. But suddenly, due to a corporate cutback, his job was in jeopardy. He found it more and more difficult to pay attention to eating right and more and more difficult to justify taking time for exercise. His weight began to creep up until he had gained back all of the weight he'd lost.

These three people are victims of backsliding. They had all made a commitment to change their eating habits and had all been successful. But then something came along or they experienced some change that encouraged them to revert to their old habits. Within a short period of time they were back where they started, only worse because they now had to contend with the fact of failure.

Most dieters have experienced backsliding. It's such a common phenomenon that unless you're prepared for it, your chances for long-term success are dismal. But ironically, the more committed you are to your new lifestyle and the greater your success has been, the more trouble you will have handling a slipup. You'll simply feel worse, blame yourself more, and may find it even more difficult to get back on track. Being prepared for backsliding could make the ultimate difference in your diet future.

On the other hand, the Maximum Metabolism Diet is unlike any other diet you may have tried: It minimizes your chances of backsliding. That's because this diet actually changes the way your body works. Maximum Metabolism frees you from the cravings and hunger that used to contribute to backsliding in the past. Not only that: After a few weeks on this diet, you'll be a different person leading a different life. You may not believe it before you try it, but eating the Maximum Metabolism way will actually change the way you think about food. It's happened to my patients and it will happen to you. You'll no longer hear the siren song of chocolates and other sweets. You'll no longer be severely tempted by fatty foods. As Lisa told me: "The thought of eating fried chicken with a large piece of apple pie à la mode now makes me feel queasy. And eight months ago it would have sounded like heaven."

Despite these great advantages of the Maximum Metabolism Diet, it's still important for you to be prepared for backsliding. You may be the kind of person who thinks a piece of your own wedding cake is backsliding and, if that's the case, you need to know how to handle whatever your future might hold.

THE 90-DAY MILESTONE

Most lapses occur in the first three months of a diet, so if you have managed to stick to your new habits for 90 days, your chances for long-term success are greatly increased. As I've said, by the time you've followed the Maximum Metabolism program for three months, you'll be a different person. You'll look different, of course, but much more importantly, you'll feel different. You'll trust yourself more. You'll have the confidence of success and your body will be your ally rather than your enemy.

I tell my patients to mark the "90-Day Milestone" on their calendars. Once they pass it, they can congratulate themselves: They've achieved a significant goal. This doesn't mean that your efforts will be over after 90 days. It simply means that you should be extra alert *during* those first 90 days of your new lifestyle.

RISKY BUSINESS

Your first slip will be your biggest challenge. If you handle a first slip successfully, you're much more likely to be able to recover from future slips. But if your first error leads to total collapse, you'll find it much more difficult to get back on track.

Backsliding doesn't happen in a vacuum. There's always a reason. In the examples I gave at the beginning of this chapter, Joan was seized by what I call an "overwhelming compulsion." She saw and smelled a favorite food and it was as if her mind shut down. She could think of nothing but eating that food. Any rational argument that she could have made against eating those cookies was beside the point. If you experience an overwhelming compulsion in the middle of the desert, you would be able to handle it. But if the smell of warm cookies triggers the compulsion and you're standing near a cookie store with a pocket full of change, you're in a dangerous situation.

Lucille was talking herself into being bored with her new lifestyle. She wanted the "variety" of a treat now and again and she was tired of the same old exercise routine. She was pleased to have the extra time that came with skipping her exercise.

Jack was experiencing a real stress. His energy was diverted into coping with his job situation and it seemed just too difficult and demanding to continue to control his eating habits.

Compulsions, boredom and stress: These are common risk situations that can encourage you to backslide. Sickness is another. If you've ever fallen off a diet when you got the flu and never resumed your diet, you've seen how sickness can sabotage a new lifestyle. Suddenly you have a wonderful excuse for not eating right, for not exercising. And to make things worse, when you're sick everyone urges you to pamper yourself.

Social situations are another high-risk area for dieters. In fact, they're such a difficult area that I've devoted an entire chapter to them. Suffice it to say here that they can be a major factor in backsliding.

THE ROAD TO HELL . . .

Some instances of backsliding are really not backsliding at all. They're the kind that usually occur after the 90-Day Milestone. You're at a dinner party and you decide to try a small piece of the chocolate truffle pie for dessert. You are not making any excuses for yourself; you're simply in the mood to taste the pie. You know that a very small piece will not ruin your diet because you have every intention of sticking to it in every other regard. This is not really a lapse; it's the beginning of "real-life dieting." If you enjoy the pie and then resume your healthy habits immediately afterward, you'll have demonstrated that you're in control of your eating.

But there's another lapse that constitutes real backsliding. It's what I call a "red-alert lapse." It's easy to recognize: When you know in your heart that the lapse is an excuse to go off your diet, that's a "red-alert" lapse. A red-alert lapse is the kind that demands strict attention and energy to survive.

What's the first thing you do after and sometimes even before a red-alert lapse? You rationalize. You rationalize that what you did was good or right or necessary or important. You don't say "I want to go off my diet because I don't care if I'm fat and it really doesn't matter to me to be thin." No. You focus instead on whatever will help you explain your action to yourself in the most acceptable way: "I'm so bored with eating the same thing every day that I'm getting depressed." "I'm under so much stress that no one could expect me to continue to pay attention to my diet." "I'm still feeling the effects of last week's cold, after all, and it's probably better for me to eat whatever I feel like eating because my appetite is so quirky right now."

As soon as you find yourself making excuses about why you had a slip, you must immediately become your own best friend. You must examine your excuses in the cold light of day. This is an aspect of the positive self-talk that we've discussed in Chapter 8 "The Inner Game of Dieting." Why did you really have a cookie binge? Why did you really start to have desserts last week when you'd skipped them for six weeks? Were you really feeling that sick or were you just looking for a rationale for skipping exercise class yet again?

You must be honest with yourself. Remember that *you* are in charge and *you* are making a decision about your future. Decisions cannot be blamed on your spouse or the weather or the fact that they were out of shrimp at the fish market so you had to have barbecued ribs for dinner. Make a concerted effort to see your motivations clearly. Some people feel tempted to test their strength after they've dieted successfully for a time. Others don't think they're losing weight fast enough and use that to justify giving up. Some people tell themselves that it's just too much trouble to prepare special diet food rather than pick up a take-out meal that happens to be loaded with fat and sugar.

Most people are very creative and convincing when it comes to making excuses to stop dieting. They know themselves well enough to realize that a weak excuse will make them feel bad, so they come up with something that surely shifts the blame elsewhere. It doesn't matter that they will soon feel bad anyhow because they know in their heart what they've done: All they want is the door marked EXIT so they can go back to their old, familiar eating patterns. Because, after all, it's not easy to change your life and it's not easy to get used to living with a stranger: a thin you.

Joan was a perfect example of this: "I guess I had spent so many years as a fat person that I was used to being treated as one. But when I lost thirty pounds my life really changed. I was going out more; meeting interesting people and people were reacting to me differently. It really sort of scared me. I was used to hanging back and passing hors d'oeuvres at parties, not conversing with strangers. And friends wanted to fix me up on dates. It was too much for me to handle and I began to eat again. It started slowly and only after I'd gained back three pounds did I realize what was happening. I really think it took courage to keep losing weight but I can tell you, once I got back in the groove I felt great. I was so proud. Before I was sort of dieting with my fingers crossed, hoping things would work out. But after that first slip I knew that nothing could stop me because I was really making it happen for myself and I was going to be able to handle the new me. And now, fifty pounds later, I can promise you that nothing tastes as good as thin feels!"

SELF-RESCUE

Once you consciously realize that you've been backsliding or once you've experienced an interruption in your diet program, you know what must be done. You have to reaffirm your commitment. But before you can do that you have to believe in your heart that one mistake is simply that—a mistake. I've said it before but I can't emphasize it enough: A slip doesn't matter; it's how you react to the slip that matters!

If you can bounce back and resume your healthy new lifestyle after a slip, you are probably well on your way to permanent weight loss.

But how do you make yourself get back on track? One of the most effective techniques is to get down in black and white exactly why you're dieting. Sometimes you really do lose sight of your goal and this weakens your resolve. Force yourself to sit down and quickly jot down a few notes. Make lists under these headings: WHAT I DON'T LIKE ABOUT DIETING; WHAT WILL HAPPEN IF I STOP DIETING; WHAT I WILL GAIN FROM DIETING.

Here's what Loretta's lists looked like:

WHAT I DON'T LIKE ABOUT DIETING:
 I don't like to avoid snacks
 I miss eating sweets and especially ice cream
 I get tired of having to think about dieting

WHAT WILL HAPPEN IF I STOP DIETING
I will have to go back to wearing my "fat" clothes
I will feel bad about myself
I won't look attractive

WHAT I WILL GAIN FROM DIETING
I'll feel in control of my life
I'll be able to wear nice clothes
I'll feel like a real success

Loretta says that she could have thought of more things for each list, but these were the things that came immediately to mind. Loretta explained the point of the lists perfectly: "Once I saw the real facts of life as far as my diet was concerned, I realized that the things I was giving up and the things I didn't like were far outweighed by the benefits of sticking to my diet. There was just no way I could rationalize that eating sweets was more important than feeling good about myself and looking good. I knew all these things in the back of my mind, but I had never organized what really mattered to me. I keep those lists pinned to my refrigerator door. They work better than all the fat-lady pictures and funny quotes I used to use to try to make me stop eating. They're *my* reasons for not eating; not someone else's."

INTERRUPTIONS

Sometimes you are actually interrupted in your diet. Perhaps you are on vacation and can't get the appropriate foods. Or you may be visiting someone. Or you may find that having houseguests for a week forces you to make a choice between being hospitable and sticking with your diet and exercise program. You simply can't expect to sail through these experiences without difficulty. It's going to take extra effort.

Perhaps the most common interruption is illness. You should stick to your diet when you're sick. It's a healthy diet and provides all the nutrients you need for a fast recovery. Just be sure to drink extra fluids and rest. You shouldn't push yourself to exercise when your body is using its resources to combat illness. But you should be able to do some exercise, even if it's absolutely minimal, unless you're completely bedridden.

These kinds of interruptions are not your fault. The trick is to recognize that the interruption is a temporary affair. You will be able to weather the interruption and stick to your diet by planning ahead. If you're expecting guests, plan meals that you can enjoy that follow your diet guidelines. Make reservations at a restaurant you know serves your kind of food. If you're flying, call the airline and order the fruit plate. If you're a houseguest, call in advance and explain your diet. If your manner is relaxed but you're firm about your goals, people won't mind. You must think of such occasions as interruptions in your *schedule*, not your *diet.* The real challenge is to recognize when the interruption is over: Some people can have a "houseguest hangover" for a month as they gobble up leftovers! It's too easy to fall back into your old eating patterns, so when you find yourself making excuses for your behavior that don't really convince even *you*, it's time to work on your own "self-rescue."

THE END?

What is the most common question asked by my patients after I describe the broad outlines of the Maximum Metabolism Diet? "When can I eat normally again?" It all depends on what you mean by "normal." The normal American diet can mean a heart attack by the time you're forty. The normal American diet means you're eating ten times the sugar you should be. The normal American diet means you're a caffeine addict. The normal American diet is killing you as well as making you fat!

From now on, Maximum Metabolism should be your normal diet. Many of my patients have told me they *want* to stick with their new eating habits. The only change I suggest is that once you reach your target weight, you can occasionally add a starch—a potato, pasta, etc.—at dinner. Of course, there will be times when you'll have some ice cream or a steak or a piece of chocolate. But when you do, it will be as a different person—not the overweight person who was once a victim of constant hunger and cravings. You'll be prepared to eat like a thin person. You'll be able to indulge in these foods occasionally without slowing your metabolism and without falling victim to a binge. You will have achieved Maximum Metabolism!

Dear Reader,

I hope that you're now on the Maximum Metabolism program and experiencing real success.

I *know* that you can lose weight. But I also know from the countless weight-loss groups and seminars I've sponsored that you're going to need help. And I'd like to give you *continuing* help and support. That's why I'm inviting you to receive—without charge— six months of my Maximum Metabolism Newsletter.

This newsletter is a monthly update for Maximum Metabolism dieters. It includes support not only from me in the form of medical updates but also from other Maximum Metabolism dieters who, like you, are facing the demands of daily life with new eating goals. I think you'll find their tips, recipes, and personal experiences will be the kind of encouragement that makes Maximum Metabolism the diet that changed your life.

If you're interested in receiving the newsletter, please write to me at the address below.

And good luck!

Sincerely,

Robert M. Giller, M.D.

c/o G. P. Putnam's Sons
200 Madison Avenue
New York, NY 10016

SOURCE NOTES

page 24 "Although it would seem . . ."
Nash, Joyce D.: "Eating Behavior and Body Weight: Physiological Influences." *American Journal of Health Promotion*, Winter 1987, 5–15.

page 28 "For example, one study found that . . ."
Nash, Joyce D.: "Eating Behavior and Body Weight: Physiological Influences." *American Journal of Health Promotion*, Winter 1987, 5–15.

page 29 "In an experiment conducted by Judith Rodin . . ."
Rodin, Judith: "Taming the Hunger Hormone." *American Health*, January/February 1984, 43–47.

page 29 "In an experiment reported in *American Health* . . ."
Rodin, Judith: "Taming the Hunger Hormone." *American Health*, January/February 1984, 43–47.

page 42 "In fact, researchers have demonstrated that . . ."
Ernsberger, Paul: "The Death of Dieting." *American Health*, January/February 1985, 29–33.

page 44 "Recent research done by Gallup . . ."
Mothner, Ira: "Our Low-Energy Eats." *American Health*, October 1987, 58–59.

page 44 "As a University of Alabama study recently demonstrated . . ."
Verner, Gayle: "More Food for Dieters." *American Health*, January/February 1984, 31.

page 45 "A recent study of overweight women . . ."
Stockton, William: "Exercise Gains Support as a Key Ingredient in a Weight-Loss Plan." *The New York Times*, March 28, 1988, C10.

page 52 "As a recent *New York Times* article says . . ."
Brody, Jane: "Scientists Find Complex Cause of Human Appetite." *The New York Times*, November 12, 1988, C1.

page 55 "Recent studies have demonstrated . . ."
Brody, Jane: "How Diet Can Affect Mood and Behavior." *The New York Times*, November 17, 1982, C1.

General References

Anderson, R., Polansky, M., Bryden, N., et al.: "Effect of Chromium Supplementation on Insulin, Insulin Binding and C-Peptide Values of Hypoglycemic Human Subjects." *American Journal of Clinical Nutrition,* 1985, 41:841.

Barnett, Robert: "Why Fat Makes you Fatter." *American Health,* May 1986, 38–41.

Blume, Elaine: "Do Artificial Sweeteners Help You Lose Weight?" *Nutrition Action Health Letter,* 1987, 14:4; 1–6.

Braitman, L., Adlin, E., Stanton, J.: "Obesity and Caloric Intake: The National Health and Nutrition Examination Survey of 1971–1975." *Journal of Chronic Disability,* 1985, 38:727–732.

Brody, Jane: "2 New Studies Point Strongly to Low Metabolism Rate as Cause of Obesity." *The New York Times,* February 25, 1988, 1–B5.

Brownell, Kelly: "Behavioral, Psychological and Environmental Predictors of Obesity and Success at Weight Reduction." *International Journal of Obesity,* 1984: 8:54–550.

Kolata, Gina: "Your Hungry Brain." *American Health,* May/June 1983, 45–49.

Morgan, Brian: "The Control of Appetite." *Nutrition and Health,* Volume 7:6, 1986, 1–7.

Saks, Peter V.: "Understanding Obesity." *The Nutrition Report,* July 1985, 52–53.

Schwartz, R., Ravussin, E., Massari, M., et al.: "The Thermic Effect of Carbohydrate Versus Fat Feeding in Man." *Metabolism,* Volume 34, 3 (March 1985), 285–292.

Tagliaferro, V., Cassader, M., Bozzo, C., et al.: "Moderate Guar-gum Additional to Usual Diet . . ." *Diabetic Metabolism,* 1985, 11:380–385.

Walaberg, J., Mathieson, R., Ruiz, K., et al.: "Effect of Carbohydrate Content of Hypocaloric Diet Plus Exercise Program on Metabolism and Exercise Capacity." *Medicine and Science in Sports and Exercise,* 1985, 17:242.

INDEX

223